HOW TO SECURE A PLACE IN MEDICAL SCHOOL

An Essential Guide for Success

I0807473

Siva Thanthullu & Thanthullu Vasu

tfm Publishing Limited, Castle Hill Barns, Harley, Shrewsbury, SY5 6LX, UK
Tel: +44 (0)1952 510061; Fax: +44 (0)1952 510192
E-mail: info@tfmpublishing.com; Web site: www.tfmpublishing.com

Editing: Dr. Christine Graham PhD
Editing, design & typesetting: Nikki Bramhill BSc (Hons), Dip Law
Cover photo: © iStock.com
Credit: Claudia Ayuso Ramirez; stock illustration ID: 1467843556

First edition:	© 2026
Paperback	ISBN: 978-1-913755-61-4
E-book editions:	© 2026
ePub	ISBN: 978-1-913755-62-1
Web pdf	ISBN: 978-1-913755-64-5

Printed by Gutenberg Press Ltd., Gudja Road, Tarxien, GXQ 2902, Malta
Tel: +356 2398 2201; Fax: +356 2398 2290
E-mail: info@gutenberg.com.mt; Web site: www.gutenberg.com.mt

Contents

Preface

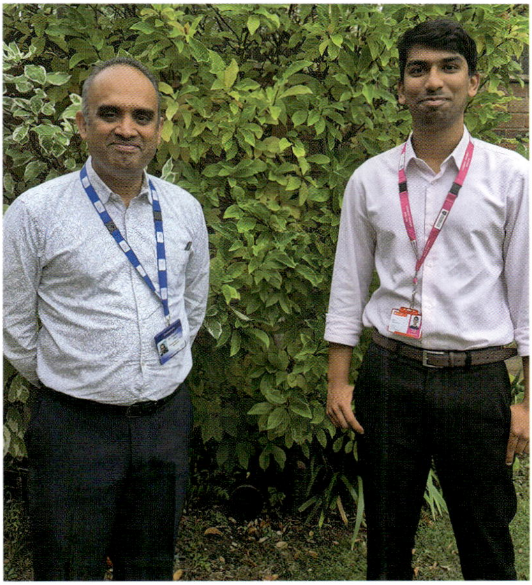

Securing a place in medical school is competitive and it can be a stressful experience for both students applying for a place as well as for their parents. Students at GCSE and A-level stage will come across lots of new terms and concepts such as the UCAT test, UCAS application, predicted scores, MMI interviews, conditional offers, insurance choices, secure offers, clearing, etc. This can be daunting, especially whilst preparing hard for their GCSEs/A-levels.

There is an average of 15 to 20 applications for each medical school place. At the same time, there are significant numbers of medical students who leave the course in the middle of their university life due to various reasons.

Universities and medical schools have a huge responsibility to make sure that they select the right candidate who can withstand the long, tiring journey of a medical career, be reflective, and cope with the stresses. To achieve this, they have to ensure that the candidates selected are not only academically highly performing, but also understand all the facets of a medical career and have the ability to cope with the pressures.

Each medical school has a slightly different selection process and varying criteria, although the overarching principles remain the same. Some place more importance upon certain criteria: for example, a part of the UCAT test called the SJT (Situational Judgement Test), while others do not; some might place importance on GCSE performance and have a scoring system during their shortlist, while others do not; some might have a maths/calculation station in the MMI, while others do not. These are just a few examples; candidates must look in detail at these criteria while selecting their universities. There is no general rule that applies to all schools; candidates must make an informed decision when choosing a school based on their own previous and predicted achievements.

This book has tried to simplify the understanding of this complex process. We suggest that candidates and parents read this well in advance so that they can start planning ahead; however, please note that universities and medical schools may change the criteria and selection process to a slight extent every year as the competition gets tougher. We advise candidates and parents to prepare as per our guidance with this limitation in mind. It is important to check the website of each medical school with regard to their eligibility and selection process before shortlisting the four universities on the UCAS application system.

Siva Thanthullu is a third-year medical student and has recent personal experience in crossing these hurdles. He has also gained experience in running various courses and advice sessions for A-level students. Thanthullu Vasu has founded and organised a national medical MMI interview course and has more than two decades of experience in helping and mentoring GCSE and A-level students towards medical careers. Both authors have also contributed to and written a textbook on MMI interviews, *Interviews for Medical School: Multiple Mini Interview (MMI) Practice* (ISBN 978-1-913755-32-4, tfm publishing Ltd, 2023), which is a useful text for interview preparation.

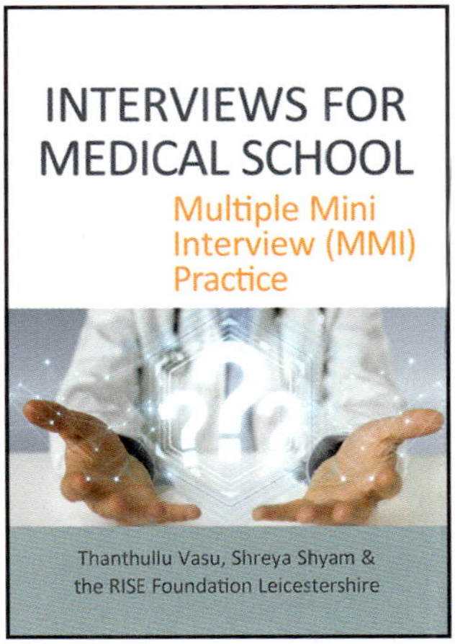

We thank Nikki Bramhill, Christine Graham and the team at tfm publishing Ltd who have worked tirelessly to publish this book; without their hard work and support, this would not have been possible. Nikki has constantly motivated us at the start of this concept, and has fully supported us throughout the whole process. We have enjoyed writing the book and really hope that this will be of use to you in achieving your dream of securing a place in medical school. We wish all our readers great success in this quest and a happy and prosperous career in the future.

We thank you for reading this book and please do send any comments and thoughts to us to consider in our future endeavours.

Siva Thanthullu
3rd-year medical student, Leicester Medical School
University of Leicester, UK.

Dr Thanthullu Vasu
Consultant in Pain Medicine and Lead for Clinical Fellowship Programme,
University Hospitals of Leicester NHS Trust, Leicester, UK.
Founder and Organiser, RISE National MMI Medical Interview Course, UK.

Abbreviations

A&E	Accident and Emergency
AI	Artificial intelligence
A-levels	Advanced levels (qualification obtained after Year 13 in the UK)
BBC	British Broadcasting Corporation
BMAT	BioMedical Admissions Test (discontinued now)
BSc	Bachelor of Science
BST	British Summer Time
COVID-19	Coronavirus disease of 2019
CPD	Continuing professional development
CV	Curriculum vitae
EPQ	Extended Project Qualification
GAMSAT	Graduate Medical School Admissions Test
GCSEs	General Certificate of Secondary Education (obtained after exams in Year 11 in the UK)
GEM	Graduate entry medicine
GKT	Guy's Hospital, King's College Hospital, and St Thomas' Hospital (medical school of King's College London)
GMC	General Medical Council (UK)
GP	General practice
ID	Identity
MCAT	Medical College Admission Test
MedSoc	Medical Society
MLA	Medical Licensing Assessment (UK)
MMA	Multiple mini assessment

MMI	Multiple mini interview
MSc	Master of Science
NHS	National Health Service (UK)
OXFAM	Oxford Committee for Famine Relief (British-founded confederation of 21 independent non-governmental organisations, a charity)
PLAB	Professional and Linguistic Assessments Board
SJT	Situational Judgement Test
SQA	Scottish Qualifications Authority
UCAS	Universities and Colleges Admissions Service (online portal for undergraduate applications in the UK)
UCAT	University Clinical Aptitude Test
UCLAN	University of Central Lancashire
UKMLA	United Kingdom Medical Licensing Assessment
USMLE	United States Medical Licensing Examination
WRVS	Women's Royal Voluntary Service

Chapter 1

Introduction to a career in medicine

A career in medicine will be extremely rewarding if you understand the training pathway, the nature of the job, the positive and negative aspects of the career, and reflect on your own attitude towards a career as a doctor. Most young students aiming to become doctors are very motivated and will have done their research before taking the step of applying to a medical school. This book will help both students and their parents to understand the pathway and prepare in the right way.

Opportunities as a doctor

If you have not had previous experience in the healthcare field, there can be many myths and misconceptions, as most perceptions about a career as a doctor come from social media and TV soaps. Medicine is a wide, diverse specialty ranging from acute medicine such as emergency medicine to chronic specialties in the community; from hospital medicine to family medicine/general practice; from clinical specialties to non-clinical specialties; from regular contact with patients such as acute medical or surgical specialties to specialties with less patient contact such as radiology or public health; and from pure clinical fields to research and management fields. In summary, there is a huge number of diversification of subspecialties, and this book cannot cover everything. Even for a medical student, it may take a few years after joining a medical school to understand whether they like medical, surgical or any other specialty; it may take some time after their graduation to further decide their subspecialty.

Length of training

Medicine has a long training period and you should be prepared for this. This duration varies between different countries in the world; the post-graduation training period varies depending on the country, and further varies depending on the specialty.

Usually, a candidate spends 5 years in a medical school for education; during the 5 years of medical school training, the candidate may get access to different types of training, including classroom-based teaching, problem-based learning, anatomy learning by dissection or prosection, and clinical teaching. They usually have to pass exams every year to progress to the next level.

After finishing medical school, the candidate goes through a period of foundation training or internship depending on the country. In the UK, foundation training is a 2-year programme to gain experience in various medical and surgical specialties after finishing medical school. The candidate acquires registration to practice after 1 year of this foundation training.

At the end of the 5-year training, they will need to pass their final year exams. Some countries have further exams before their registration with the medical council to allow them to practice. In the UK, the candidate has to pass the United Kingdom Medical Licensing Assessment (UKMLA), which tests their core knowledge, skills and behaviours, before they can practise; furthermore, there will be a separate assessment of their prescribing skill. In the USA, the United States Medical Licensing Examination (USMLE) three-step exam will be the way forward after medical school.

Once you complete the medical school and foundation training, you may want to do postgraduate specialisation; this can vary from 4 to 10 years depending on the specialty and the country. Acute clinical specialties take 2 years of core training and 5 years of specialist training after medical school in the UK, whereas, the general practice pathway can last for 4 years after medical school in the UK. Doing American Board exam training might be shorter than this, but it will be more intense training with longer hours per week; it usually takes a 3–6-year residency programme to specialise in the United States.

Lifelong learning

A doctor should be committed to lifelong learning. Medicine constantly evolves; new inventions in technology and the discovery of new medications are the routine. To practise safely and successfully, the doctor should keep themselves up to date on these new changes. Furthermore, to keep themselves revalidated for their practice, they have to show evidence that they are keeping their skills, knowledge and expertise regularly updated by various continuing professional development (CPD) courses or training. Professional development for a doctor is an ongoing journey that continues throughout the time that they practise in the field of medicine.

Work–life balance

Some specialties in medicine might require working long hours or working unsociable hours (such as night shifts); a candidate interested in medicine should be aware of this. The authors recommend that interested candidates should have done observership or work experience in a healthcare-related field and be aware of the different clinical fields within hospital medicine and general practice/family medicine before applying to a medical school. However, this problem is not unique to medicine alone; a person in other non-medical specialties such as banking, investment and entrepreneurship could also work during unsociable hours.

Why select a career in medicine?

Medicine can be a highly rewarding career for motivated candidates with the right expectations. A doctor is directly involved in impacting the lives of patients. A doctor will treat pain and illness at the most difficult times of their patients' lives. Even today, being a doctor is a highly respected profession with the public. A survey conducted a few years ago in 35 countries showed that doctors topped the global list of the most respected professions, with a score of 11.6 out of 14.

A doctor is still one of the top earners in society; opportunities to progress in their specialty and career are possible. Furthermore, some doctors diversify into different careers including education/teaching, medical management, entrepreneurship, pharmaceutical industry, research, medical journalism, medicolegal work, etc.

The job of a doctor can be intellectually stimulating and happy; working in a team, working in crisis situations, and resuscitating a very ill patient can all create satisfaction and happiness. Even comforting a terminally ill person or a person with difficulties will lead to a patient thanking the doctor, which can give a huge morale boost and be satisfying to the doctor.

According to a recent BBC survey, doctors have topped the list of jobs that teenagers want to do when they are older; this increased recently after the pandemic and has been at the top for the last 2 years in 2024 and 2025. In the UK, the National Health Service (NHS) was the top organisation preferred by teenagers in which to work when they get older.

What are the pitfalls in a medical career?

The ideal profession for a candidate depends on their individual interests, attitudes, skills and values; this could also vary depending on their personal circumstances. As discussed earlier in this chapter, a doctor's job can be stressful and will involve working long and unsociable hours. There is a proportion of doctors or medical students who leave their career as it can be exhausting for them. Being prepared and understanding how to maintain a good work–life balance is the key to success in a medical career.

For an aspiring doctor, it's important to talk to various healthcare professionals and observe/shadow them to understand the pros and cons of the profession before taking the step of applying to medical school.

Key Points

- **A medical career has lots of opportunities, with diverse specialties within it.**
- **A career in medicine can have a long training period, depending on the specialty.**
- **A medical career is well respected and can result in good financial rewards.**
- **Medicine involves lifelong learning.**
- **A career in medicine can be stressful, especially if the challenges are not met.**

References

1. BBC Bitesize. Revealed: New entry in top 10 jobs teenagers want. Available from: https://www.bbc.co.uk/bitesize/articles/zrfknk7.
2. World Economic Forum. 10 most respected professions in the world. Available from: https://www.weforum.org/stories/2019/01/most-respected-professions-in-the-world/#:~:text=Best%20&%20most%20respected%20professions%20in,government%20managers%20and%20management%20consultants.&text=Librarians%20fared%20even%20worse%2C%20consigned,list%20may%20look%20quite%20different.

Chapter 2

Are you the right person to be a doctor?

Young teenagers doing their A-levels or GCSEs may be puzzled about what career might suit them well. It is a difficult decision and they need to do adequate research, not just about the particular career, but whether their inherent values, qualities and attitudes will fit well with the profession. Medicine has huge diverse specialties within it, but still there are some common qualities that need to be present before choosing this career. This chapter describes some of these desirable qualities; the reader can reflect on whether their values match with them before selecting their career.

Compassionate and empathetic person

Sympathy involves feeling sorry for another person's difficult situation without necessarily sharing their emotional experience. Empathy is the ability to understand and share the feelings of another person; it involves putting oneself in another person's shoes and experiencing their emotions and feelings. Compassion is more than empathy, as you not only put yourself into the shoes of others, but you also do something about it by taking action. In the interviews, most medical schools test to ensure that they are selecting candidates who display compassion and empathy.

Research has shown that compassion can improve patient satisfaction, quality of care, and physician effectiveness. The General Medical Council

(GMC), which regulates doctors and provides a licence to practice, emphasises compassion as a core professional standard for doctors. In the *Good Medical Practice* guidance, the GMC stresses that doctors should treat patients fairly and respect their rights; they should be kind, courteous and respect their patients (Domain 2: Patients, partnership and communication).

Communication skills

Communication is more than just providing information; it has a vital role in establishing good rapport and relationships with the patient and their family. This will ensure the safe delivery of high-quality healthcare. Doctors also need communication skills to work with other multidisciplinary colleagues in a team.

Most complaints against doctors are due to communication issues; most medical schools test the communication skills of candidates who apply for a place via their multiple mini interview stations.

Active listening is a key skill for healthcare professionals. Listening to a patient's concerns and their preferences is important in forming a good management plan.

Teamwork

Modern healthcare systems are complex and need good teamworking skills to have the best outcome. Working together with other members of the team to provide coordinated care is vital. It is important to value the role of each member of the team and respect them.

Critical thinking and problem-solving skills

Doctors are intelligent and adapt themselves to complex working situations. Complex medical situations need good problem-solving skills to make sound decisions. Many medical schools use situational judgement testing (SJT) (see Chapter 9) to test these skills before selecting them for the medical school.

Honesty and trustworthiness

Doctors are well respected in society and patients trust them with their lives; the GMC expects an important level of personal and professional standards of conduct for doctors and medical students (see Domain 4: Trust and professionalism, *Good Medical Practice*).

Organising skills and time management

Doctors should be punctual and well organised; the medical profession can be demanding with a busy workload. Keeping accurate records and documentation are essential for doctors.

Resilience

A doctor's job can be demanding and stressful. Resilience is the doctor's ability to adapt and manage these stresses and adversities. Doctors should have good coping strategies, have a good work–life balance, and should seek help when needed. When applying for medical school, it is important that the candidate has awareness of these issues as these will be assessed in the interviews.

Medical Schools Council statement on core values

The Medical Schools Council agreed on the core values and attributes needed to study medicine and published guidance in 2018. The applicants should be motivated to study medicine and show a genuine interest in the medical profession; this is tested in the interview and the personal statement. Having insight into their own strengths and weaknesses is the key to reflecting on themselves as a doctor. They should be conscientious and take responsibility for their own actions.

Reflecting on yourselves

It is advisable for those interested in a medical career to ensure they have the attributes to match the above-mentioned qualities; students at their GCSE/A-level stage should conduct extensive research to make sure they are selecting the right career. It may be worth analysing if they can demonstrate these qualities from their real-life experience, which may not be necessarily related to the healthcare setting. If they feel they have the qualities, it may be worth reflecting on how to improve these skills while considering an application to medical school.

Key Points

- **There are core values and attributes needed to be a doctor.**
- **Being compassionate, empathetic and having good communication skills help to build a good rapport with patients and their families.**
- **Honesty and trustworthiness are essential for a doctor and a medical student.**
- **It is important that a candidate applying to medical school reflects on these qualities and uses their real-life experiences to demonstrate them.**

References

1. Aynsley-Green A. The case for compassion. British Medical Association. Available from: https://www.bma.org.uk/news-and-opinion/the-case-for-compassion.
2. British Medical Association. Good communications as a medical student; June 2024. Available from: https://www.bma.org.uk/advice-and-support/ethics/medical-students/ethics-toolkit-for-medical-students/good-communication.
3. General Medical Council. Good medical practice. Domain 2: Patients, partnership and communication. Available from: https://www.gmc-uk.org/professional-standards/the-professional-standards/good-medical-practice/domain-2-patients-partnership-and-communication#:~:text=Treating%20patients%20with%20kindness%20courtesy%20and%20respect&text=You%20must%20treat%20patients%20with,a%20cure%20may%20be%20possible.
4. Medical Schools Council. Statement on the core values and attributes needed to study medicine. 2018 update. Available from: http://www.medschools.ac.uk/media/2542/statement-on-core-values-to-study-medicine.pdf.
5. Uygur J, Brown JB, Herbert C. Understanding compassion in family medicine: a qualitative study. *Br J Gen Pract* 2019; 69(680): e208–16.

Chapter 3

Introduction to medical schools in the UK

There are approximately 50 medical schools in the UK. There may be slight changes in the curriculum, teaching strategies, and the structure of the programme, but most of them offer similar competencies. These are guided by the GMC's requirements for the licence to practise. All assessments from these medical schools are structured to make the doctors competent with the domains of *Good Medical Practice* and give them the skills and knowledge needed to progress towards the foundation programme.

If a candidate wants to become a doctor, any of the medical schools in the UK will serve this purpose; furthermore, recent changes in allocation to the foundation programme mean that the candidate may end up moving far from the medical school once they finish the 5 or 6 years of study.

Each candidate might choose a medical school based on various factors, including the teaching technique used, curriculum, city where the school is located, presence of medical societies and facilities to continue their hobbies, reach of outdoor pursuits, etc. It is important to visit open days run by the medical schools in order to get a feel on how the school aligns with your values and passions (see Chapter 7).

The requirements for admission vary for each medical college to a small degree; these are covered in Chapter 12.

In the following section, we have listed colleges that focus on undergraduate courses in medicine (code A100); there are also new schools opening up. Websites and contact details are published in Chapter 12.

Medical schools in the London area

The medical schools in the London area include:

- University College London Medical School.
- King's College London GKT School of Medical Education.
- Queen Mary University of London, Barts and The London School of Medicine and Dentistry.
- Imperial College London School of Medicine.
- City St George's University of London.
- St Mary's School of Medicine, Twickenham (only international).
- Brunel University Medical School (only 50 UK students, others international).

Medical schools in the south of England

The medical schools in south of England include:

- University of Bristol Medical School.
- University of Exeter Medical School.
- University of Plymouth Peninsula School of Medicine.
- University of Oxford Medical School.
- University of Southampton School of Medicine.
- Brighton and Sussex Medical School.
- Kent and Medway Medical School.
- University of Cambridge School of Clinical Medicine.
- Norwich Medical School, University of East Anglia.
- Anglia Ruskin University School of Medicine.
- University of Surrey Medical School (opened in 2025).
- University of Buckingham Medical School (only private with fees).

Medical schools in the Midlands

The medical schools in the Midlands include:

- University of Leicester Medical School.
- University of Birmingham Medical School.
- University of Nottingham School of Medicine.
- University of Lincoln Medical School.
- Keele University School of Medicine.
- University of Warwick Medical School.
- Aston University Medical School.
- Three Counties Medical School, University of Worcester (opened 2024 entry).

Medical schools in the north of England

The medical schools in the north of England include:

- University of Liverpool School of Medicine.
- University of Manchester School of Medical Sciences.
- University of Sheffield School of Medicine.
- University of Leeds School of Medicine.
- Newcastle University Medical School.
- University of Sunderland School of Medicine.
- Lancaster Medical School.
- Hull York Medical School.
- University of Central Lancashire School of Medicine & Dentistry.
- Edge Hill University Medical School.
- University of Greater Manchester Medical School.
- University of Chester School of Medicine.
- Pears Cumbria School of Medicine.

Medical schools in Scotland

The medical schools in Scotland include:

- University of Glasgow Medical School.
- University of Edinburgh Medical School.
- University of Aberdeen School of Medicine.
- University of Dundee School of Medicine.
- University of St Andrews School of Medicine.

Medical schools in Wales

The medical schools in Wales include:

- Cardiff University School of Medicine.
- Swansea University Medical School.
- Bangor University, North Wales Medical School.

Medical schools in Northern Ireland

The medical schools in Northern Ireland include:

- Queen's University Belfast School of Medicine.
- Ulster University School of Medicine.

Chapter 12 details the requirements and entry criteria for each medical school listed above and provides links to their website. Each candidate may have different strengths to fit the requirement criteria; Chapter 13 explains how a candidate should select their choices for the four medical schools while applying to the UCAS.

Key Points

- **There are more than 40 medical schools in the UK.**
- **The candidate applying to medical schools should be aware of the details of the school and what it offers to students.**
- **Open day visits will help the candidate to understand more about the medical school, the university, and the city of residence.**

References

1. Medical Schools Council. Medical Schools A–Z. Available from: https://www.medschools.ac.uk/for-students/applying-to-medical-school/medical-schools/.

Chapter 4

Stages in the preparation for medical school

Once you have decided to apply for medical school, it is essential to understand the various stages that a candidate will be involved in when preparing for this application. This book will discuss each stage separately in the following chapters; this chapter will just provide an overall summary of the pathway.

■ Figure 4.1 overleaf shows a schematic diagram of all the stages in the medical school application process.

GCSE level

Many students at GCSE level may feel that it is too early for them to decide on a medical career or any other career. Please remember that most medical schools (not all however) include the GCSE scores for shortlisting for the interviews (see Chapter 12). It is essential that the student decides at Year 11 if this is the right career path for them, and starts working towards it. It is ideal to get at least grade 6 or more in at least six subjects, including English Language. Further details are discussed in Chapter 5 in this book.

Stage	
Decision	Research the career; compare your values. Decide on medicine as your career. Discuss with professionals, observe and reflect.
GCSE	Aim for a grade 6 or more, in at least six subjects. Select science subjects. English Language might be essential.
A-levels	Predicted grades are important in Year 12; at least AAA is quoted by many schools. Chemistry is important and Biology might help for the future. Aim for A*AA as a minimum.
Experience	Work and voluntary experiences will help. If you can't get a health-related experience, then use an allied experience in other fields, which might be acceptable.
UCAT	Prepare for at least 4 months in Year 12; aim to take the UCAT in mid or late August. Online practice experience is useful. Aim for at least 2100 in three components in total, with SJT band 1.
UCAS	Your personal statement must be your reflection; be truthful. Choose from four medical schools; this should be based on your GCSE scores, your UCAT scores and the requirements of that particular medical school.
Interviews	Multiple mini interviews are used in most schools — preparation is the key. Do a lot of role-play practices before the interview. Try to demonstrate and reflect on your work experience in the interview questions.
Selection	One sure choice and one insurance choice in June. You should achieve the needed grades, either AAA or A*AA. Results day in August might be stressful; be prepared.

Figure 4.1. Schematic diagram showing the stages in the medical school application process (please see the following chapters for further details; this is an overall summary of the pathway and exceptions apply).

A-levels

A-levels in Years 12 and 13 will be very busy; a candidate aiming for a medical school place should be motivated to work hard. They should work in Year 12, aiming to achieve good predicted grades (AAA as a minimum, but the authors recommend A*AA); these predictions will be given in most schools in July in Year 12 or later. This is needed for filling in the UCAS application, which will be done in October in Year 13. The break between Year 12 and Year 13 will be busy with UCAT exam preparation, in which the candidate should aim for at least 2100 or more out of 2700, with an SJT banding of 1.

Year 13 will continue to be busy with UCAS applications in October, and interviews from December to March; the candidate's anxiety levels can rise as they expect interviews, attend interviews, and wait for the results. The candidate still has to continue with their school academic preparation to make sure that they achieve the required minimum grades in the final exam in Year 13. If you are lucky and are offered places in medical schools, you will finalise your first choice and insurance choice in June in Year 13 while taking the final A-level examinations. The anxiety will continue until the results day in the middle of August after Year 13. A-level preparation is further detailed in Chapter 6 in this book.

University Clinical Aptitude Test (UCAT) exam preparation

The UCAT is one of the most important steps in the pathway to enter a medical school; many students may not give the right attention and time to this step and fail miserably. Having awareness of this exam and preparing in the right way helps in securing an interview at the medical school. Most candidates prepare for 4–5 months at the end of Year 11; it is prudent to work hard to get the scores to fit the selection cut-off criteria for the interviews. If your UCAT score is low, when applying to the UCAS, you need to select the medical school that places less importance on this test. Some medical schools will select only SJT band 1 for interviews (despite mentioning the minimum criteria as SJT 1, 2 or 3); this needs to be kept in mind when applying on the UCAS system as you would have received your scores. For details on the UCAT exam, please refer to Chapter 9.

Preparing for the interview

Interviews can be stressful; if a candidate has prepared well in advance, it will be easier to succeed. Most of the schools have moved to a multiple mini interview (MMI) pattern, which standardises and removes bias among the examiners. We recommend reading our textbook *Interviews for Medical School: Multiple Mini Interview (MMI) Practice* (tfm publishing Ltd, 2023; ISBN 978-1-913755-32-4), which contains 133 different scenarios (all author royalties from the sale of this book go to charitable causes). We also recommend the RISE MMI course run annually in November in Leicester, which provides real mock scenarios for MMI interviews. This course is fully run by volunteers, organised by the RISE Foundation Leicestershire charity; again, the money goes to charitable causes (details are available on the website: https://risefoundationuk.com/mmi/). See Chapter 14 in this book for more details on how to prepare for the interview process.

Coping with the pathway

This process of preparing for medical school can be daunting or overwhelming for some; this book will help to provide candidates with the necessary knowledge so that they can approach the task with confidence, and ensure that they are preparing to face these hurdles in the right way. We suggest taking a good break after finishing GCSEs and recommend having a break of 1–2 weeks after the UCAT exam before the school restarts for Year 13.

■ Figure 4.2 outlines the timeline in the preparation process for medical school.

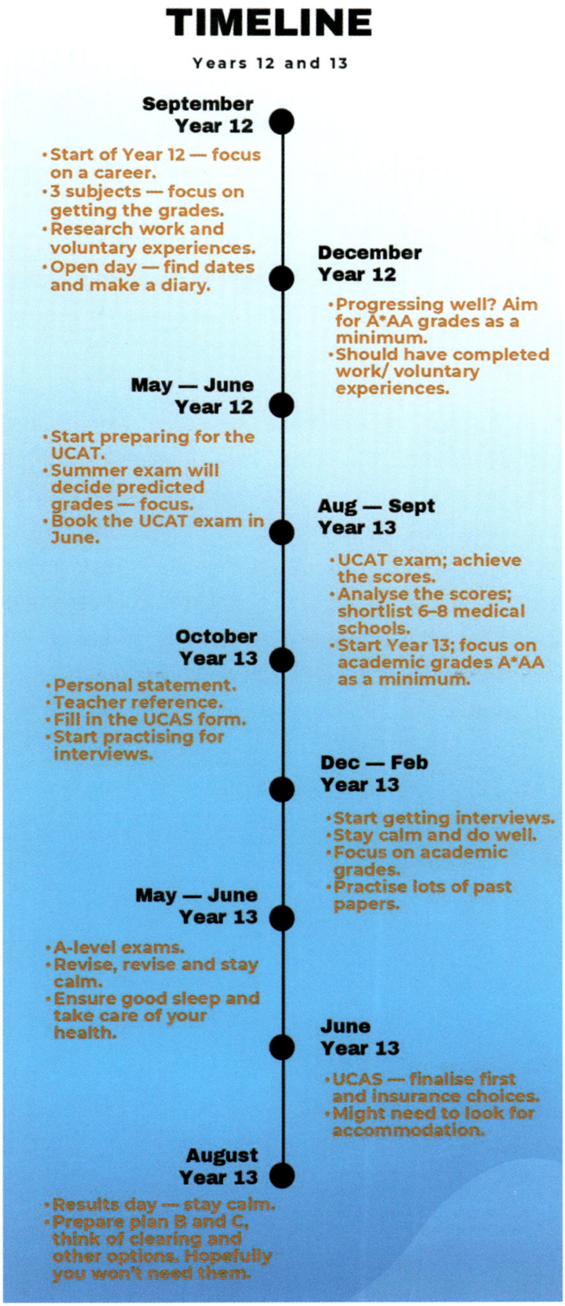

Figure 4.2. Timeline in the preparation process for medical school.

Taking care of physical and mental health

The difficult task of preparing for medical school occurs during the teenage years when there may be lots of distractions. Some students can become overwhelmed and we recommend taking care of their health while they engage in this process.

Taking care of their physical health by regularly visiting a gym, playing a sport, or engaging in any other hobby to maintain their fitness levels is vital. Eating a good nutritious diet is also important.

Mental health takes more priority as these steps can be seen as significant hurdles by many students; the stress levels can rise during each of these steps, including predicted A-level grade exams, UCAT exams, applying for universities, waiting for news about interview invites, attending the interview, waiting for results, preparing for the A-level exams, and finally facing the results day. Having a good social set-up is essential during these times to support oneself. Getting a good sleep of at least 6–8 hours per day will help a lot in this process. See Chapters 21 and 22 for details on how to take care of physical and mental health.

Key Points

- **There are various stages in the preparation for applying to a medical school.**
- **A candidate should start focusing from GCSE levels; getting good grades in A-level exams is vital.**
- **UCAT exam scores and GCSE grades help in securing an interview.**
- **GCSE, UCAT and interviews are the major hurdles, while getting A-level grades will make them successful in securing a place in medical school.**

References

1. RISE MMI interviews. Available from: https://risefoundationuk.com/mmi/.
2. Vasu T, Shyam S, RISE Foundation. *Interviews for Medical School: Multiple Mini Interview (MMI) Practice*. Shrewsbury, UK: tfm publishing Ltd; 2023.

Chapter 5

Preparation at GCSE level

We recommend that students make a decision at GCSE level on whether a medical career is the right choice for them. Many medical schools take the GCSE score into consideration before inviting candidates to an interview; most but not all schools give a 40–50% score for the GCSE grades for interview selection.

Making a decision in the GCSE years

Years 10 and 11 are vital foundation blocks for a student aiming for medical school. Not only do these years give them the basic knowledge of the academic subjects, but they also make them think of various careers and how their inherent values, attitude, skills and knowledge will fit into the right career. Schools usually hold career days and career sessions with the aim of exposing students to a wide range of careers; GCSE students should utilise these opportunities, and talk and liaise with people from all different careers. Some schools will have career advisers who carefully study the particular student's profile and their achievements and make recommendations for the future.

If you are interested in medicine as a career, you should be showing motivation to pursue this from the GCSE years. Talk to your form tutor or lead teacher as they have the experience to guide you on the right path.

Selecting subjects for GCSEs

If you are interested in medicine, you should select and focus on the sciences (Chemistry, Biology and Physics), English Language and Mathematics. Most medical schools require a minimum of grade 6 in at least six subjects to apply for medicine; however, it is wise to still achieve higher grades than a 6 as many universities score according to your grade and take this as an approximately 50% total score for the selection criteria for the interviews. Given the huge competition in the application of medicine (a minimum of 15–20 applications for each place in a medical school), candidates are advised that the best chance of success is by getting a grade of 8 or 9 in six GCSE subjects, although this is not compulsory. Many schools want English Language and Science to be compulsory in these six subjects.

Science subjects

Science provides the basic foundation of medicine; most exam boards have the option of either triple science or combined science. Triple science has three separate GCSEs, in Biology, Chemistry and Physics; this covers more topics in depth and has longer exams. The authors recommend triple science as this gives them a better foundation to proceed towards medicine. Chemistry is compulsory for many medical schools; it gives a basis of how the body works, how medications and chemical reactions in the body function, and provides a good understanding of the basics of medicine. Biology teaches the knowledge of the body parts and their functions. Physics will help to understand the body mechanics and the various types of equipment that are used in medicine. Triple science or separate sciences will get you three separate GCSEs while combined science or trilogy will get you only two GCSEs. Combined science gives a broader overview and covers less depth; the exams are shorter in duration and depth.

There is no restriction on which science subject you should take at GCSE level for entering medical school; even taking combined science will be acceptable. Even to do A-level science, having a GCSE in science is not a prerequisite or restriction. However, the authors recommend triple science to gain a better and broader understanding of the science subjects before entering medical school.

Mathematics

Many medical schools recommend having a basic knowledge of mathematics; it helps doctors with problem-solving skills. A basic knowledge of mathematics helps in the calculation of drug doses, the estimation of chemical reactions in the body, the use of different technologies in monitoring and treatment, and in research and statistics. This is not compulsory but some medical schools have a station of basic calculations, statistics and data analysis in one of their MMI stations during the interview. A few medical schools also have a mathematics paper as a basic requirement before proceeding to the interview. A student has the choice of looking at the requirements of the medical school and applying accordingly based on their strength and weakness analysis. The UCAT exam tests basic knowledge in mathematics and can be easier with studying mathematics at GCSE level (see Chapter 9).

English Language

Most medical schools require the candidate to have English Language in their GCSEs. It helps the schools to assess their communication skills, as this is vital in the everyday practice of a doctor.

Other subjects

Most schools or colleges have a foreign language as a requirement at GCSE level; medical schools may consider this an advantage. Having Music, Art, Food Tech, PE, etc. can help if this can be explained in the interview to demonstrate their extra-work passion and skills; this will make the interviewer confident that the candidate takes care of themselves and can cope with stress in their future career. This is not asked as a requirement by the school, but if the candidate is intelligent, this can be expressed in the interview to gain good 'brownie points'.

Subject choices

In the end, the best choice depends on the student's personal interests; there are exceptions to the guidance given above as some of the universities differ in their requirements. The student should research their own strengths and weaknesses, and discuss their options with their teachers and the career guidance staff; the teachers and guides will analyse the student's personal wish regarding careers, their goals and the motivation to achieve them, their track record of performances in the past at school and advise accordingly. If you differ from their advice, then it is wise to discuss why and explain what steps you can take to rectify the deficiencies that have been quoted. A motivated student can work hard to achieve what is required. The guidance mentioned in this book covers the general rules based on most medical schools, but there are always exceptions to these.

Please note that medical schools vary in requirements; some may be strict with the subject choices, while some are flexible about GCSEs. It is prudent to check with the specific entry requirements of the particular medical school that you are interested in (see Chapter 12). There is always the option to look at different choices of medical schools depending on your strengths. However, achieving high-level grades in GCSEs gives you a variety of options for applying to medical schools.

Summer schools

It is difficult for the under-16s to get work experience, but any voluntary experience related to the healthcare sector might help. Further details are available in Chapter 8.

Some medical schools run summer schools that provide introductions and taster days for medical schools. For example, Brighton and Sussex Medical School runs a BrightIdeas programme, and a 4-day summer school for students when they are in Year 12. The attendees do research on a chronic condition of interest and then explore, report, share and reflect on this concept. Oxford runs a summer medicine course for those aged 15–18.

Key Points

- **It is prudent to decide on a career while doing GCSEs.**
- **Selecting science subjects and achieving good grades, along with English Language is recommended.**
- **Triple science can give a better and broader understanding to prepare for medicine as a career, rather than combined science subjects, although this is not compulsory.**
- **Many medical schools take GCSE scores for selecting candidates for interviews, but there are exceptions.**
- **Achieving high grades in GCSEs opens up many options for applications to medical schools.**

References

1. Brighton and Sussex Medical School. BSMS Virtual Work Experience. Available from: https://bsmsoutreach.thinkific.com/courses/VWE.
2. Medical Schools Council. Entry requirements for 2025 start. Available from: https://www.medschools.ac.uk/studying-medicine/how-to-apply-to-medical-school-in-the-uk/entry-requirements.

Chapter 6

Preparation at A-level

A-levels in Years 12 and 13 can be very busy for a student preparing to apply to medical school. There are three vital stages in this process (see timeline in Chapter 4, ■ Figure 4.2), namely:

1. Getting predicted grades from Year 12 assessments.
2. UCAT examination at the end of Year 12.
3. Medical school interviews.

The students will be busy not only due to these three stages, but also with other additional processes in these 2 years, including work and voluntary experience, attending university open days, preparing the personal statement, applying through the UCAS application service, and making sure that they work hard in Year 13 to achieve good grades. Some of these are discussed in the following chapters in this book. We strongly advise students to focus and work hard, but at the same time take care of their physical and mental health; ensuring good nutrition and adequate sleep are vital in order to continue the pace of work during these 2 years.

Keeping focused during the A-level years

If a student is interested in applying to medical school, they should let their school or college know about their ambition. Their form tutor or head of the year will be supportive and can guide them through this challenging pathway. If there is an opportunity to get involved in the medicine, science or biology clubs in their school/college, it will help in networking and learning about the available opportunities. Many schools/colleges will guide students through the UCAS applications with special modules and study sessions nearer the time of submission of the application. The student's teacher will need to provide a reference for their UCAS application; it will help if students have liaised with them from the beginning and discussed their progress and challenges.

Selecting subjects for A-level

For A-level, we suggest selecting three subjects that include Chemistry and Biology; the third subject could be Mathematics or Physics, but there are also a huge number of other options. If you want a fourth subject, the Extended Project Qualification (EPQ) may be an option. Concentrating on three subjects and getting a minimum of A*AA is recommended, although there are many other ways to succeed also.

Chemistry is important as most medical schools have it as an essential requirement. Having Biology A-level is required by many medical schools, but this can be exempted in a few schools. If you have both Chemistry and Biology A-levels, it opens up the option to apply to a wide variety of medical schools. Furthermore, Chemistry and Biology provide a solid foundation to work with when the candidate enters medical school.

Mathematics may help, as some medical schools have calculations and statistics as part of their interview stations, but GCSE-level knowledge may be enough. Having mathematics is not compulsory. Knowledge of mathematics can help the candidate when they enter medical school as it helps when understanding drug and physiological calculations and concepts.

Many medical schools accept a variety of options for the third subject; many students select Physics, Psychology, History, Geography, Social Science, and modern language subjects. Many medical schools do NOT accept subjects such as General Studies, Critical Thinking and Citizenship studies. It is wise not to select related subjects such as Mathematics and Further Mathematics together among the three subjects in A-levels. It is important to check with the medical school requirement criteria for the preferred university, researching whether the subject is acceptable before planning the selection of A-level subjects.

Having an EPQ as the fourth subject may open up the option of application for some universities such as Lancaster if a lower grade is achieved in one of the three subjects (e.g. AAB). However, this is only available in a handful of medical schools. The downside is the time needed for the preparation of this fourth subject.

We recommend three A-level subjects; Chemistry and Biology are the best subject choices as they open up the option of a wide variety of medical schools to apply to; the third subject option can be Mathematics, Physics or a subject of the candidate's choice in which they have a huge interest. They should aim to achieve grades of A*AA as a minimum in these three subjects.

Extended Project Qualification (EPQ) as a subject

An EPQ is an optional project done in Year 12 in most schools or colleges; for some medical schools only, this can compensate if a grade drops below the minimum required in the other three subjects. An EPQ can be on any health-related topic based on a written dissertation, audit and research, or a model or artefact made with the aim of promoting health. The scoring is based on the reflection of their thoughts and the work done for the project. An EPQ helps to assess the student's motivation, organisational skills, hard work in researching health-related topics, self-directed learning and, finally, presentation skills.

We recommend only three subjects and aiming to achieve grades of at least A*AA; if a candidate is not confident in achieving this, an EPQ may be an option, but their options for medical school are limited in this case. As this can compromise the time available to study in the other three subjects, spending that time to achieve A*AA grades in the core three subjects may be wise, but this depends on the personal capacity of the student.

Researching medical schools

It is vital that a candidate and their parents conduct suitable research on the medical school, the university and the place/location of the school before deciding on their choices. While conducting research, it is vital that they read the minimum requirements for the medical school application and assess if the candidate's criteria fit with the requirements. See Chapter 13 for more details.

Many medical schools will publish the previous year's selection cut-off criteria; this will give students an idea of how they will fare in the selection to that medical school. It is essential that you pick 6–8 universities that you might like and then deep dive into the research based on the minimum criteria and the previous year's cut-off. For example, a particular university might publish that the minimum criteria is a grade 6 in GCSEs, AAA in A-levels, and a particular UCAT score; whereas if you look at last year's selection cut-off in the same university, it will say that the majority who got selected had a grade 8 in GCSEs, A*AA in A-levels, and a SJT score of band 1 rather than 2 or 3 mentioned as a minimum in the UCAT scores. You should know where you stand with all these requirements at the beginning of Year 13; while applying to the UCAS in the month of October in Year 13, be prudent and do not waste choices without doing the research.

Keeping busy with A-levels

While Year 12 goes very quickly with settling into college or school and understanding the basics of the three subjects, you may have to work hard to get the predicted grades at the end of Year 12. Year 13 continues quickly with analysing your UCAT scores, preparing the UCAS application, visiting open days, etc.; within 3 months of the start, you may get stressed with invitations to interviews (from the end of November). The next 3 months (December to

February) will be occupied by interviews for the four medical schools to which you have applied. By the time you receive a conditional offer in March to May, you will have only a few weeks to prepare for the final A-level exams and make sure that you achieve the grades that are the minimum for this offer. These steps look overwhelming at the outset, but the school will prepare and support you through them; if you have enough knowledge of this pathway, this can feel easier. This book discusses all these steps in separate chapters that follow for easier understanding.

Preparing for A-level examinations

The schools and colleges offer regular academic feedback on the performance of candidates in every term of A-levels; these should be taken seriously and actively reflected upon. Most of the time, these teachers' allotted grades/score predictions are right and their serial reports tell you how you are progressing throughout the year. Many schools and colleges not only give a grade based on the work of the candidate, but also a score for the effort that they are putting in; the effort shows whether they could do more or whether it should continue in the future. A trend of the scores in these assessments from Year 12 is vital; when the candidate reaches Year 13, it is vital to check that these are maintained and are in line with the needed minimum grades in final A-level examinations. Also, an upward trend can allow teachers to give a good predicted grade after Year 12.

Practising past exam papers for A-level examinations

While each candidate may have their own way of preparing for the examinations, it is vital to practise past papers for each subject; these will be available from their exam boards. Rather than reading textbooks alone, these past papers will help the candidate to assess their performance and reflect on it. This is a very important step in the preparation as the exam assesses the practical application of a concept rather than reading the theory itself. The exam boards also specify how they scored the past papers; this will give an idea on how a student should answer a particular question.

Other tricks for A-level exam preparations

Each person has a different way of preparation but a few suggested tricks by past candidates include:

- Having a timetable for preparation and actively reflecting regularly on this timetable on progress.
- Using flashcards to revise for exams; stationery shops or online shops sell standard flashcards that you can write on and use to revise.
- Ready-made published flashcards for subjects are available, but we recommend that candidates make their own for revision.
- Understanding what the exam is assessing is vital; applied knowledge of a concept is important at A-level.
- Engaging actively in a class, not falling behind, organising well, and mastering the content are needed. Studying for A-levels is a continuous process for the 2 years and students should use a strategic plan that is reflected on regularly.
- Regular revision, revisiting the topics, and consolidating your knowledge help in the examination.
- There are a huge number of online resources that are free; if you do not understand a concept in a textbook, try to research online and understand it before proceeding further. At the same time, stay focused as online access can be distracting.
- Strong regular study habits and sufficient time to take care of your physical and mental health, are important; good sleep and nutrition are vital.
- If your well-being is affected, seek help early; without your health, you cannot achieve success however hard you work.
- A positive mindset improves outcomes; stay motivated. Talk to your teacher and career adviser if you are behind in this.
- We feel that stress is inevitable during the busy A-level years; proper relaxation techniques and staying motivated help to manage the stress.

Exam techniques for success

The A-level exams start in early May and run through until the end of June in Year 13. Each subject has three papers and a candidate needs to stay focused. If you feel that you have not done well in one paper, do not lose your concentration; it will also have been difficult for most other candidates. It is worth focusing on preparing for the remaining examinations and keeping up the motivation.

It is vital to understand the objectives of the assessment in these tests; reflect on the mark schemes to make sure that you are answering what the exam question specifically asks. Make sure you answer all questions in the exam paper; managing time effectively and appropriately (as per the score for each question) can help. If a candidate has answered many past exam papers (in exam conditions), this will become easy in the final examination.

Exam day preparation

You should have prepared and revised well in the last 2 years and there is no point in getting stressed at the last minute. Try to get a good night's sleep before the exam. Have a good breakfast and practise relaxation breathing strategies on the morning of the exam (if you have used them before). Organise what you need for the exams on the night before the exam. Try to go to the exam venue early and try not to talk about the topics with others just before the examination, as this can stress you.

Once the exam paper is given, work through it in a calm and structured way. Read the question thoroughly to make sure you understand what that particular question is assessing. Work your time effectively to answer all the questions. If there is remaining time, go through the paper once again to make sure that you have not made any simple mistakes.

Getting stressed does not help in exams. You have worked hard up to your potential in the last 2 years; remember this and keep yourself motivated. There may be some tough and difficult questions in each exam, but stay focused and do your best.

Key Points

- **A-levels in Years 12 and 13 can be very busy for a candidate preparing for medical school.**
- **Three vital steps include: getting predicted grades, getting good scores in the UCAT exam, and doing well in the interview.**
- **Selecting three subjects that include Chemistry and Biology opens up a variety of options for medical school entry.**
- **Exam preparation techniques are vital; organising yourself, staying focused, and revising regularly help in this preparation.**
- **Practising past exam papers is a vital step to scoring high grades in A-level examinations.**

References

1. British Medical Association. Applying to medical school. Nov 2024. Available from: https://www.bma.org.uk/advice-and-support/studying-medicine/becoming-a-doctor/applying-to-medical-school.

Chapter 7

Attending open days at universities

Before selecting a medical school option, a candidate may want to visit open days at some medical schools to explore their programme, curriculum, campus and the city itself. A student at a medical school will spend the next 5 years in this university and the city; it is vital that they research well before entering the medical school. Attending open days is not compulsory; but the medical schools expect the candidate to have done some research about their school, curriculum and city before applying. This knowledge will help at the interview stage but this does not necessitate attending an open day.

What is an open day?

All medical schools have open days that provide A-level students with an experience of visiting their campus, teaching facilities and living conditions, and have some volunteer senior students showing them around the campus. A few medical schools also have some lectures organised to show what the teaching and the subject will look like. This open day is meant to attract the candidates to their medical school, but the students and parents should use this opportunity to analyse if their goals and ambitions will be fulfilled by that particular school and its curriculum, as well as the opportunities available in the city.

Pattern of the open day

The pattern of the open day varies between different universities. Some even run virtual open days rather than in-person days. Usually, medical schools have regular dates, mostly during the summer and autumn. The dates and details are available on the websites of each university.

Programme and curriculum

Medical schools vary in their curriculum and the way it is delivered; the common structures include traditional teaching, problem-based learning, integrated teaching, case-based learning and module-based learning. Some medical schools teach anatomy by dissection of cadavers, while most use prosections. Each candidate has their own liking for the learning technique and these open days can be useful to research and analyse these learning techniques.

Campus tours

Some medical schools will want you to book a particular time for the tours that run throughout the day. The campus tour gives the prospective students a flavour of the facilities available such as the library, classrooms, lecture halls, anatomy dissection halls, laboratories, gym and sports facilities, and student accommodation. These are usually run by current students who have settled well in the university; this experience can help prospective students understand the culture and environment that they are going to enjoy for the next 5 years.

Social activities, including MedSoc (various societies for activities) groups, will be advertised during these open days; these help the candidate to analyse if they can practise their hobbies and passions while being at the university.

Meeting staff and students

It will be a good opportunity to meet the staff who may discuss the facilities and other opportunities including that of research. The staff can advertise the success story of the university and the medical school during these sessions. Students will be volunteering in different parts of the campus, and also advising and guiding the prospective candidates.

Selection process

Some medical schools have a session on how they select candidates; these sessions can help the candidate to clear their doubts about whether their scores/grades will be sufficient to enter the medical school. They will answer questions on their cut-off scores, interview pattern, etc.

Special sessions, workshops and modules

Some medical schools run special workshops or modules (such as anatomy stations, simulation exercises, hands-on workshops, or on using medical devices, etc.) to attract prospective students.

Q&A sessions

The open day will have various opportunities to answer the questions of both candidates and parents.

Should I attend the open day?

While attending an open day can be helpful, some candidates may be stressed whilst applying to medical schools and shortlisting at least 6–8 schools; time may be an issue. Most open days are also available on recorded videos through online and social media platforms. There are also discussion forums on various social media platforms. Attending the open day is not compulsory, but it can help you to better understand what to expect at a particular medical school.

During the interviews, it is prudent to show that you have done enough research about the university, medical school and the city. This will provide confidence to the interviewer that the candidate is motivated and focused. Some MMI stations focus on why the particular candidate has applied to this medical school; it is vital to prepare the answer to this question in various domains such as the curriculum, learning technique, city for living, etc.

It might be possible to visit the open day in Year 12, as the applications need to be done in the early part (October) of Year 13. This saves further stress during the busy period in Year 13 with both academic preparation and UCAS application preparation.

How to plan for an open day

The authors advise looking at the website of the medical school/university and planning ahead to also help streamline their A-level preparation. Once you have shortlisted 6–8 universities, it is worth going to their websites and checking if you fulfil the minimum requirement criteria and fit the selection cut-off from the previous years. Then, create a diary looking at the available dates for open days from these universities. Attending two or three may give you a flavour for these open days, but make sure that you are focused at the same time on your A-level preparation.

Checklist for open days

A candidate may want to check the following questions during the visit for open days:

- Do I like the medical school?
- Do I like the university campus and facilities?
- Do I like the city?
- Do I like the student accommodation?
- Do I have opportunities to continue my hobbies or passions?

- Does the school have good student support and social life?
- Is travelling between hospitals and the medical school easy? Where should I go for hospital/GP surgery postings?

In addition, it is vital to research:

- What is the curriculum and programme?
- What type of learning/teaching does the school have? Does it suit me?
- What clinical facilities are available in this school?
- What type of anatomy teaching do they have? Dissection or prosection?
- Are there facilities for research, intercalated degrees, etc. if you want them?
- How do the existing students feel about their medical school?
- What exam or assessment techniques does the school use?

Key Points

- **Open days in medical schools/universities can provide valuable insight about the curriculum, learning techniques, clinical facilities, social life and the city.**
- **Attending an open day is not compulsory, but it is helpful to experience the university and the medical school where the student might be spending the next 5 years.**
- **Prepare a checklist before you go to the open day and feel free to ask questions to address your doubts.**

References

1. British Medical Association. Applying to medical school. Nov 2024. Available from: https://www.bma.org.uk/advice-and-support/studying-medicine/becoming-a-doctor/applying-to-medical-school.

Chapter 8

Work and volunteering experience

Work experience and volunteering experience are important to secure a place in a medical school. Medical schools expect the prospective candidates to be motivated and have an understanding of the work involved in the medical field; work experience can help to prove that you have these qualities, including the right attitude, values and behaviour. Most candidates do have these experiences, but fail to demonstrate them in their interview answers; it is also important to reflect on how these experiences will help in your future career. Although clinical or healthcare experience is desirable, some candidates may find it difficult to obtain this experience. Relevant volunteering experience or part-time work can be accepted, provided the candidate is intelligent enough to show the transferable skills to a medical career and demonstrate their motivation towards medicine.

What can work experience deliver?

Before planning a lifelong career, a student should have some understanding of the profession and find out if their attitude and values will align with the profession. Working in the healthcare sector needs motivation and an empathetic attitude. A period of work experience in a hospital, care home or a GP setting will give a reasonable understanding of the medical field for a candidate; it will help them to reflect on whether they can cope with the pressures of the job and assess their ability to interact with patients in care. Furthermore, work experience can motivate some students and help them work hard in academic subjects to reach their goal. Medical work experience can be very rewarding for A-level students when they see difficult scenarios and how the healthcare team has tackled them. The authors can quote many examples in which A-level students have reflected actively, such as observing a complex surgery, a doctor discussing a terminal illness, seeing modern technology in medicine, working as a team in an operating theatre, etc. These situations may help the candidate to decide if medicine is the right choice for their future.

Healthcare-related work experience

Health and care work experience can be attained in various ways:

- Hospitals may have work experience posts for A-level students; enquire about the hospitals in the region to find out the availability. There might be an application system to make sure that the paperwork on confidentiality and patient safety is taken care of. Usually, the hospitals give a one- or two-week observership for this purpose under a named clinician.
- GP or community centres. GP surgeries may have provision for observation but again you need to contact a few nearby surgeries in advance and check the protocols for this. If clinical shadowing is not available, it is worth asking for observership in administrative roles, such as helping or observing clerical and administrative staff, which can aid the candidate in getting an understanding of the system.
- Care homes can offer work experience for short- or medium-term periods, especially at care homes for older people. It is worth enquiring about nearby care homes in advance.
- Pharmacies can offer placements that can help with learning about medication; it also provides an opportunity to communicate and liaise with patients.
- Physiotherapy, diagnostic services, midwifery, and other allied professions can also offer valuable placements in the healthcare system.

Voluntary or community organisations

Various voluntary or community organisations can offer placements both in clinical and non-clinical settings; these experiences can be reflected on in the medical school interviews. Organisations such as OXFAM, the British Heart Foundation, cancer charities, the Women's Royal Voluntary Service (WRVS), the Red Cross, St John Ambulance, etc. often have shops or outlets where volunteering can also be done.

How to find a work or volunteering experience

This should be planned well ahead, starting when a candidate is 16 years old. Most establishments only allow work when the candidate enters Year 12. Schools and colleges often have career guidance departments, which may have a list of establishments offering work or volunteering experiences. It is advisable for any candidate to start enquiring well in advance, with the appropriate preparation in order to demonstrate their motivation. A brief CV and reason for the observership might help these establishments in deciding on the possibility of an observership or a volunteering experience.

Universities and medical schools may offer shadowing or observer experiences and it is worth researching the availability of such experiences in nearby universities. If you do not succeed in your search, liaise with your school career advice team or teachers who can direct you in the right way.

For volunteering, various organisations such as the Scout Association, Girlguiding UK, Sea and Air Cadets, St John Ambulance, etc. may have opportunities. You could also enquire with nearby foodbanks or animal rescue centres if that interests you. Some charities may give you an opportunity to help with fundraising or organising activities. Working in a charity shop may help, but the candidate should be prudent enough to reflect on the transferable skills and use the available opportunities for their future career. Good communication skills, being empathetic, and a willingness to help others are key attitudes in any work or volunteering experience for a candidate interested in a medical career.

Virtual work experiences

The COVID pandemic changed the way in which observership or work experiences are done, as virtual work experience is now also available. It is worth searching for these opportunities to see if they will be useful for you.

Some establishments run weekend online work experiences with various team members of the health service; these could be useful for understanding how the NHS works and how it relies on teamwork.

The Royal College of General Practitioners runs an online platform called Observe GP, which is an interactive platform with eight videos; this explains all about the GP practice, including the receptionist, administrative side, as well as the clinical aspects. It is free and available to anyone in the UK who is 16 years old or above.

Some medical schools themselves deliver virtual work experience with lots of useful modules. For example, Brighton and Sussex Medical School has a virtual work experience and this can be accessed online; it involves an introduction followed by six specialist areas that provide insight to the candidate. This course is strongly recommended if you are applying to this medical school; even if you are applying to different medical schools, this will be a positive addition to your personal statement or demonstration in interviews.

How long should the work experience be?

There is no specific time limit for work experience in most of the medical schools; only a handful of medical schools ask the candidate to list the duration of their experience. Most medical schools expect to see a candidate's experience but do not question the duration or specificity. However, when the candidate writes a personal statement, it has to demonstrate their strong motivation towards medicine as a career. More importantly, the work or volunteering experience is mostly assessed while the candidate attends the MMI or panel interview stations. These interviews can either directly ask about work experience or expect the candidate to elaborate when there is a related question, even if it has not been asked explicitly. For example, if the interview station is about teamwork, the candidate can volunteer that they have seen how teamwork was important when they observed it in a particular clinical or volunteering setting from their own experience; this may add extra marks for that station. In another example, if the examiner asks why communication skills are important for a doctor, the candidate can volunteer in their answer that they have seen a situation in which they realised the importance of communication from their clinical work experience. Personal examples from their work or clinical or volunteering experience add much to the outcome of the interview stations.

However, the authors have seen many candidates who have had many months of work experience, but it was not demonstrated in the interview stations. If this is not demonstrated, then the purpose of the work experience is defeated!

We recommend doing at least 1 week each in both hospital and GP settings with some virtual experience and volunteering experience.

Duke of Edinburgh's Award experience

Many students may have enrolled in the Duke of Edinburgh's Award programme; this allows the candidate to do a variety of volunteering experiences, which can be correlated to the medical field while answering interview questions. In the skills section of this award, a candidate may have learnt a new skill; this can be helpful in demonstrating motivation, teamwork, and other aspects such as taking care of themselves. In the interviews, rather than saying that they have done a particular Duke of Edinburgh's Award, the candidate should reflect on how these skills can be useful and transferable to a career in medicine. The Duke of Edinburgh's website provides guidance on volunteering and directs how to find an opportunity if any candidate is interested.

First aid and basic life support courses

First aid and resuscitation courses can be useful as a work or healthcare-related experience. St John Ambulance and other charities may offer courses for this.

Reflection on the experiences

The work and volunteering experiences serve two major purposes:

1. To determine if healthcare is the right career for the particular candidate.

2. To answer the interview questions, with a demonstration of their motivation towards medicine.

Many candidates fail in the second purpose, in that they do not take the opportunity to reflect on their experience during interviews. They may have written about these experiences in their personal statement, but it is vital to demonstrate and reflect on these experiences in the interviews.

To help in reflection, the candidate can use notes to jot down the important events during their observership; even having a separate folder on their computer to save these experiences and reflections may help later during the preparation for the interviews. These could be either happy scenarios, or even challenging scenarios in their observership; reflecting on both of these situations will help the candidate for their career in the future. Reflection helps a candidate to develop competencies, attitudes and values, and helps them to think carefully about their future career choices.

Reflective diary

Reflection helps us to think about our experiences; the GMC stresses the need for reflection for doctors and medical students.

A reflective diary helps candidates in their future career. The Royal College of General Practitioners and the Medical Schools Council have published an example of such a reflective diary, which is freely available online. It is important to document your observations and reflections as soon as possible after the work experience whilst it is still fresh in your memory.

A reflective diary has four phases:

1. Describing what happened.
2. What were your thoughts and feelings at that time?
3. Analyse what was good and what was not good about this experience.
4. How can it be different in future?

Important tasks for work experience

For work experience, the authors suggest:

- To start planning early, as it can be difficult to find work experience in some situations.
- Liaise with the providers and find the pathways.
- Prepare a short CV before you approach the providers.
- Be proactive once an opportunity is available.
- Note down some important scenarios at the end of the day; this will help you to reflect as well as use them in your personal statement or interviews.
- Reflection is the key during any work or volunteering experience.
- Thank the clinician, team and the provider at the end of the session as they are trying to help you amidst their busy work.
- The candidate gives a thank you card to the team as this will motivate them to do more for young students wishing to enter medicine.

What should you do during the work experience?

We recommend the following code for those attending their work experience:

- Be punctual, try to show your motivation, and be helpful to the team if there is an opportunity.
- Dress in a professional manner.
- Be polite, and introduce yourself as an A-level student on placement to learn before applying to medical school.
- Communicate with patients or staff when possible and learn/understand their views.
- Introduce yourself to the patient if the clinician has not done so before.
- Some patients may not want students to be there during the conversation; understand their emotions and step out. It is nothing personal, but patients are in difficult situations and you need to respect their wishes.
- Try to speak and liaise with the whole team, including the receptionist, administrators, other healthcare staff, and patients.

The NHS depends on teamwork and it is vital to be aware of and respect the roles played by all the staff.

Patient confidentiality

It is important that a candidate doing work experience respects patient confidentiality. You should not discuss patients with anyone, or on social media. The GMC takes this very seriously for doctors and medical students, and the same rule also applies for those observing the healthcare set-up. If the patient turns out to be someone you know, such as a friend or family member, it is wise to step out of the consulting room as it may be embarrassing for the patient to discuss their health problems openly in front of you.

Key Points

- **Work experience is vital to assess your attitude, qualities and behaviour towards medicine as a career; further it gives you an understanding and clarifies whether you like the profession.**
- **Volunteering experience can be useful, but you need to reflect on how these experiences will help in your medical career and how the skills are transferable.**
- **Online or virtual work experiences are available.**
- **It is vital that you demonstrate these experiences in your medical interviews and personal statement.**
- **Due to practicalities, it is advisable to start planning earlier and approach hospitals or GP surgeries in advance.**
- **Liaise with teachers and the career guidance team in school who may be able to guide and help in this regard.**
- **Remember the code of conduct while observing patients, in particular, confidentiality.**

References

1. Brighton and Sussex Medical School. BSMS Virtual Work Experience. Available from: https://bsmsoutreach.thinkific.com/courses/VWE.
2. British Medical Association. Getting medical work experience. June 2025. Available from: https://www.bma.org.uk/advice-and-support/studying-medicine/becoming-a-doctor/getting-medical-work-experience.
3. Duke of Edinburgh. Volunteering. Available from: https://www.dofe.org/lifezone/volunteering/.
4. Royal College of General Practitioners. GP work experience. Available from: https://www.rcgp.org.uk/your-career/work-experience.
5. Royal College of General Practitioners. Webinar — What is Observe GP? RCGP. Available from: https://www.youtube.com/watch?v=0BsRnl1C8G8&t=122s.
6. Royal College of General Practitioners and Medical Schools Council Selection Alliance. Inspiring and preparing tomorrow's doctors. Reflective diary. Available from: https://www.rcgp.org.uk/getmedia/02dcaf12-9cf9-4494-86db-745d422d76e8/RCGP-reflective-diary-June-2019.pdf.

Chapter 9

University Clinical Aptitude Test (UCAT)

The UCAT is a computer-based aptitude examination that is used for assessment and selection by most medical schools. It is used in conjunction with other criteria, such as academic performance. It is one of the most important parts of the application process, with most universities requiring applicants to meet a cut-off score to progress towards interviews. This chapter will briefly explain the components of the UCAT and the techniques to prepare for this examination.

It is widely thought that 'you cannot revise for the UCAT'; however, the authors are of the opinion that this is not true. Although you cannot predict the material that will arise on the test day, it is imperative to get accustomed to the format of the examination and practise as much as you can to achieve good scores. As you will learn with practice, timing is one of the most difficult components of the UCAT.

Booking a UCAT examination

The UCAT is an online examination run every year in Pearson Vue test centres throughout the UK and worldwide (it might be the same centre as your driving theory test for some candidates in the UK). More than 40,000 students take this exam every year. Booking starts in mid-June and ends in mid-September every year; check the website for the correct details. Book the test as early as possible to get the dates of your choice. Late dates might be released later by the booking system.

You will create an ID and login before booking the exam. You have to keep this UCAT candidate ID safe if needed, as it is linked to the UCAS account. Please make sure that you enter the details correctly, as the UCAT automatically sends results to the UCAS through a data-matching exercise.

UCAT format

In total, the entire examination should take close to 2 hours, and consists of four sections: verbal reasoning, decision making, quantitative reasoning and situational judgement (from 2025 onwards, the abstract reasoning subtest has been removed and is no longer assessed). All four stations have a multiple-choice format. There is no negative marking for wrong answers; you should always answer all questions, even attempting a guess, rather than leaving them blank.

It is important to note that once the test has been started, it cannot be paused and it is not possible to revisit a previous section. See ■ Table 9.1 for the structure of the examination.

Table 9.1. Structure of the UCAT examination from 2025.

Subtest	Time per question (seconds)	Number of questions	Total time (minutes)	Scoring
Verbal reasoning	30	44	22	300–900
Decision making	63	35	37	300–900
Quantitative reasoning	43	36	26	300–900
Situational judgement	23	69	26	Bands 1–4

Verbal reasoning

The verbal reasoning section consists of 44 questions. There will be 11 passages, each associated with four questions. You are given 90 seconds at the start to read the instructions, and then have 22 minutes to answer 44 questions. This equates to just 30 seconds to answer each question; each passage has 2 minutes only.

Due to the strict time constraints, the authors feel that it is not feasible to read the entire passage to start with. Instead it can be helpful to focus on the questions first, and then scan the passage, looking for any similarities that may relate to the question. This method of scanning the text can be improved by doing practice questions and mock tests under realistic time constraints.

The passages of text can be based on any theme, and are usually based on a non-academic topic. However, you will never be expected to use any prior knowledge on these topics and it is important to only use the information that is provided in the passage. Look out for implications within each passage that allow you to draw conclusions. Do not make assumptions in the absence of the given information.

The best way to improve your speed reading skills is to regularly skim news articles for key facts. Online practice courses will prepare you better and they also help you to assess your technique of answering.

There are five types of verbal reasoning questions:

1. True/False/Can't tell — the passage is followed by a question which gives you a statement and asks you if it is true or false or if you can't tell. This is only based on the information provided in the passage.
2. Incomplete statements — a statement is followed by four answer options to conclude; you choose the most appropriate answer that will finish the statement.
3. According to the passage — you will be given a statement and asked to choose which of the four answers is best supported by the passage; note that the answer option can be lengthy.

4. Except questions — you weigh up the evidence to reach a conclusion based on the information in the passage. One out of the four answers is not reflected in the passage and this is selected.
5. Most likely — based on evidence; however, the choice may appear less definite and a little more speculative.

Decision making

The decision-making section consists of 35 questions. You are given 90 seconds at the start to read the instructions, and then have 37 minutes to complete the section. This leaves approximately 63 seconds to answer each question.

This section analyses the candidate's ability to apply logic to reach a decision, evaluate arguments and analyse statistical data. Please note that the decision should only be based on the information provided and you should not use your own beliefs or biases to reach the conclusion. You may be given text, charts, tables, graphs or diagrams.

There are two formats of decision-making questions. Some will give four options, with only one correct answer. The other variety will ask if a given statement is true or false. Some questions require multiple responses; in these, 'almost right' answers can also fetch partial marks.

Students will realise that questions always follow a similar format; prior preparation is key to scoring well on the exam day.

In preparation for the decision-making section, students may find it useful to revisit the mathematics topics such as probability and practice interpreting graphs again. It can be useful to draw the information out in the form of a Venn diagram to better visualise the problems. To save time, try to solve only what is asked in each question.

This section can have the following question types:

1. Syllogisms — logical argument that applies deductive reasoning to arrive at a conclusion; these have multiple answer options; you need

to drag and drop the correct answers. Do not make assumptions and use only the information given in the question. You need to read carefully the words such as 'some', 'all', 'none', and 'only' as this will help you to come to a conclusion.

2. Logical puzzles — four answer options with only one correct one; using a grid system to write information may help. Try to rule out answers that cannot be true. Read carefully words such as 'must' or 'might'. Work out the needed answers only.
3. Recognising assumptions — evaluating arguments for and against a problem; only one correct answer; select the strongest argument.
4. Interpreting information — interpret from written passages, graphs and charts; use reasoning skills; have multiple answer options; need to drag and drop answers.
5. Venn diagrams — might ask for the best conclusion, or make you draw a Venn diagram, or ask which Venn diagram is the best representation. Only do the work needed for that answer.
6. Probability and statistical reasoning — a short passage with statistical information; select the best answer.

An on-screen calculator is provided for use in this section; there are no scientific functions in this calculator. You can practice using this calculator on the official mock tests on the UCAT website.

Quantitative reasoning

The quantitative reasoning section consists of 36 questions that need to be answered in 26 minutes. This leaves just 43 seconds per question.

Quantitative reasoning asks GCSE-level mathematics questions that evaluate the student's numeracy skills. The UCAT website states that they are testing problem-solving skills rather than numerical abilities. The questions will usually refer to charts or graphs with data. Most questions appear in groups of four and are linked to the same data, but some may be stand-alone questions and so it is important to read the questions carefully.

Focus on the question being asked rather than getting diverted by the extra information provided. Read the question carefully as individual words may be crucial. Key topics that you need to revise include:

1. Percentages, decimals and fractions.
2. Rates — speed, flow, etc.
3. Proportions and ratios.
4. Average (mean), median, mode and range.

As mentioned earlier, an on-screen calculator is provided and you should practise using this calculator on the official mock tests on the UCAT website.

Situational judgement test (SJT)

In this section, you must answer 69 questions in 26 minutes, leaving 23 seconds per question. The situational judgement section assesses your core values and how you respond to real-life situations which you may come across as a medical student and doctor. Students are not expected to have any prior medical knowledge. The SJT assesses various characteristics including: perspective thinking, integrity, team involvement, resilience, and adaptability.

Students will be presented with a hypothetical situation in a clinical or educational setting with up to six follow-up questions related to it. Some questions will give four options and ask you to choose the most appropriate ones. The other format involves ranking three options from the most appropriate to the least appropriate. It is possible to get partial marks in this section if you are close to the correct answer.

Some questions ask you to rate a response; you could use the same rating more than once or even not at all. You need to make a judgement about the answer option independent of the other questions in the scenario. You select only one response, and even if your answer is close to the correct answer, you can get partial marks. Remember to understand the meaning of the words: 'very important', 'important', 'of minor importance', and 'not important at all'.

The SJT subtest is scored differently, with students given one of the Bands 1–4. We strongly recommend candidates to prepare by reading the *Good Medical Practice* document from the GMC as it outlines the key principles required to be a good medical student and physician. It is also vital to be familiar with the four pillars of medical ethics: autonomy, non-maleficence, beneficence and justice:

1. Autonomy — giving respect to the patient and letting them make the decisions.
2. Non-maleficence — doing no harm.
3. Beneficence — always acting to benefit the patient.
4. Justice — consideration of the law and the overall benefit to society.

Computer system

Practising online for 1–2 hours for at least 4–5 months can help while you increase this duration nearer to the examination. It is important to practise using the answering system on the computer as it helps in the actual examination. It may be wise to practise using the on-screen built-in calculator rather than a separate one as this is not allowed in the actual examination.

Keep an eye on the timer in the top right-hand corner of the screen; below this, you can see the question number that you are working on at that time. Pace yourself and stay calm during the test. If a subtest has not gone well, try to clear your mind before the next subtest and do not let this affect the next subtest. Always stay positive for these 2 hours of the examination.

Getting familiar with 'Flag' and 'Review' functions in the test will help; this will help you to revisit the marked questions before finishing a subtest. If you are unsure about a question, eliminate the wrong answers and use your best judgement; you could 'flag' it for review and move on; some candidates mark 'flag' for tough questions, and move on to easier ones and come back to the tough ones and take the time that is available.

If you have time remaining at the end of the subtest, you can use the 'review' screen to go back and revisit the flagged questions.

When to sit the exam?

The UCAT examination should be taken between July and September after finishing Year 12. This score will be taken automatically by the UCAS application system for the medical school entrance. The booking system opens at the beginning of July.

The advice varies depending on when you can sit the exam; a minimum of 3–4 months preparation and practice is recommended. If you can start this preparation at the end of May in Year 12, you may be able to take it in the third or fourth week of August, which will make sure that you get a couple of weeks' break before starting Year 13 at your school or college. This break is essential as it will be very busy in your Year 13. However, students differ in the technique and preparation for the UCAT and some prefer taking it in September. The authors recommend the third or fourth week of August for the reasons explained above.

Please note that you can take the UCAT examination only once for that year. The UCAT Consortium does not advise practice runs in previous years and can take action if they find out. However, you can take the exam in the following years if you are not successful and are planning to apply again.

What time to book?

Different timing slots will be available during the booking system; it depends on your individual preference. Some might like it early in the morning, and some prefer it late. This is an examination held in an online exam centre and can get busy as the day goes on; if the weather is hot (in August), it can be tiring for the candidate if they choose a slot in the late afternoon. We recommend taking it in the morning when you are fresh, but it can vary based on your preference. Please note that there may be other exams also happening in the centre, such as a driving test or entry to different courses.

Online courses

The authors strongly recommend online practice courses, which are available for the UCAT examination. Online examination simulates real exam conditions as managing time pressure is the key to success. Practising how the exam system works on both the UCAT website and in the paid online courses will help you in the real exam. You might subscribe to these online websites for 3–6 months.

The authors recommend getting a subscription to these online courses for 1 or 2 months after the GCSE break as there will be a long gap in the summer before starting Year 12. This helps to gain awareness of the system and knowledge of how the test works. If you have this awareness, it will help later to prepare in a more focused manner after Year 12, when you take the actual examination.

General advice

The UCAT is definitely a challenging component of the application process; simple tricks can help you to achieve good scores:

- Do not leave any questions blank: all four sections of the UCAT are multiple choice, and none has any negative marking. Make sure to guess intelligently if you run out of time.
- Start revising early: we advise at least 3–4 months of preparation for the UCAT exam. There are various resources available to help you prepare. Practise the practice questions on the UCAT website; some other good online resources include Medify, Medic Portal, etc.
- Do not leave it until it is too late: although it can be tempting to book an exam slot at the end of the summer holidays and maximise revision time, later slots are busier, and will lead to a stressful start to Year 13.
- Practice under time pressure: replicating exam conditions is vital in making sure that you are prepared for the exam day.
- Use official resources: the official UCAT website has four mock tests and a question bank for all of the subtests. These are the most similar to the actual exam that you will sit, so make sure to have completed

these before your exam. It is useful to do the mock tests towards the later stages of preparation.

- Familiarise yourself with the software: make sure you know how to use the online calculator and the keyboard shortcuts to save as much time as possible.
- Do not panic: you have done the work to prepare! Do not let the exam stress you out.

On the test day

You should take an original personal photo ID with you to the test centre, such as a passport or a full or provisional driving licence in the country of issue. The UCAT Consortium advises arriving 15 minutes before the appointment time for the check-in process. The authors advise checking the car parking or travel arrangements and arriving at least 30 minutes before. You may wish to travel a few days before to familiarise yourself with car parking, etc., although you will not be allowed into the centre if you are not sitting the exam.

Apart from photo ID, nothing else will be allowed in the test room; there will be a storage area for personal belongings. Food and water are not permitted in the test room and must be stored outside.

Test centres usually accommodate up to 15 candidates, and some may be taking a different examination. You will be monitored at all times, by both audio and video which may be recorded.

You will be allotted a desk space with a computer, keyboard and mouse. You will be given a laminated A4-size notebook and a pen; an on-screen basic calculator is integrated into the test.

If you take a break in the test, you will lose time when you go out of the room as the clock will continue. If you have to take a break, it is best to take it between subtests as it may not compromise a single section heavily, but it will still compromise the total timing available.

The results will be issued (a copy of your UCAT score report) immediately after the examination; it takes up to 24 hours to update on your UCAT web account.

The test statistics will be published in mid-September; this may help you to analyse where your score is compared with others. This contains the final mean scores, deciles and percentiles.

Your UCAT results will be automatically delivered to the chosen university in early November. You do not need to pass your test results to the universities or UCAS.

Key Points

- **UCAT is a computer-based aptitude test, required by most medical schools.**
- **It has four sections: verbal reasoning, decision making, quantitative reasoning and situational judgement.**
- **Online practice is vital before going for the real exam.**
- **Time is the most crucial factor for this exam; practice makes you successful.**
- **Please take this exam seriously as these scores are the basis for getting an interview.**
- **You can only sit this exam once in the year of your UCAS application.**

References

1. General Medical Council. Achieving good medical practice: guidance for medical students. Available from: https://www.gmc-uk.org/education/standards-guidance-and-curricula/guidance/student-professionalism-and-ftp/achieving-good-medical-practice.

2. General Medical Council. Good medical practice. Available from: https://www.gmc-uk.org/professional-standards/the-professional-standards/good-medical-practice.
3. UCAT (University Clinical Aptitude Test). About the University Clinical Aptitude Test (UCAT). Available from: https://www.ucat.ac.uk/.
4. UCAT (University Clinical Aptitude Test). Question Tutorials. Available from: https://www.ucat.ac.uk/prepare/question-tutorials/.

Chapter 10

Personal statement

When you submit an application for UCAS (see Chapter 11 for UCAS), you will need to submit a personal statement. Some medical schools use it for shortlisting for the interviews, while most medical schools do not read the personal statement until the candidate is selected; rarely, if two candidates get the same scores in all sections, the statement can be used to distinguish them. A few medical schools use it in an MMI station for discussion. Personal statements should reflect the candidate's motivation towards medicine as a career, and show their work or voluntary experience for this. It is good to display your hobbies and other interests to show that you have a good work–life balance to meet the stresses of a doctor's career.

Structure of a personal statement

A personal statement should be limited to 4000 characters or 500 words only for the UCAS application; it is difficult to summarise all your qualifications, experiences, and achievements within this limit. It should include:

- Your reason for motivation.
- Experience — either work or volunteering, with a reflection on how it will help your future career.
- Your hobbies, interests, and extracurricular activities.

- Your academic and other achievements.
- Why you are best suited for medicine.

Recent UCAS changes for the personal statement

UCAS has announced that the personal statement format will be changing from one longer piece of text to three separate sections. UCAS has done this with the view that these three questions will help applicants to scaffold their answers and ensure that they include exactly what the universities want to see.

Each answer will have a minimum character count of 350 characters, which will be clearly labelled on the question boxes, with an overall character count. The 4000 overall character limit (including spaces) remains the same however.

The three questions include:

1. **Why do you want to study medicine?**

- Your motivation for studying medicine:
  - have you been inspired by a role model or a moment in your life?
  - what has driven you towards studying medicine?
- Your knowledge of this area and interests:
  - have you researched any area in medicine?
  - is there a book or subject that has sparked your interest?
  - do you have any super-curricular activities of curiosity and interest in medicine outside the classroom?
- Your future plans and why medicine fits you:
  - why is medicine your future?

2. **How have your qualifications or studies helped you to prepare for medicine?**

- Transferable skills that you gained from formal education.
- Subjects in the school or college related to medicine and achievements.
- Your strengths and achievements related to applicability for medicine as a career.

- Accomplishments and winning competitions, serving as team captain or ambassador or lead for any school clubs.

3. **What else have you done to prepare outside of education, and why are these experiences useful?**

- Work experience, volunteering or part-time employment.
- Personal life experiences and responsibilities.
- Hobbies and extracurricular or outreach activities.
- Achievements outside of school or college.
- Post-education activities if any.

Avoid plagiarism

Modern software can easily detect plagiarism; it is definitely recommended to avoid copying someone else's statement. The medical schools can easily find this out. Be honest as this is one of the most important qualities recommended for a doctor. Use your own words and write with your own emotions.

Experience

It is vital that you display your work and volunteering experience, and reflect on how it shaped or motivated you. If you have done any part-time job or summer school experience, reflect on what these will do for your medical career, and what skills can be transferred to medicine.

Why am I best suited for medicine?

You can explain your attitude and behaviour, but it should be done with evidence. You may have received some award or recognition in the health or care field. You may have done a project or written an article related to healthcare. You may have participated in a school club or community clubs related to science or health. Write it in your statement with an explanation of how you have reflected on these activities.

Hobbies and extracurricular activities

The selectors are looking for a well-rounded person who can balance work and life; a medical career can be stressful and medical schools place importance upon the physical and mental health of students. It is worth showcasing your talents or interests in hobbies, music, art, sports, etc. Rather than just mentioning that you play a sport or music, you should display your achievements and reflect on how they help you to balance yourself.

Personal life experiences

Not everyone can fill this in, but if you have had any personal experience within the health or care sector, it is worth reflecting on what these experiences did to you as a person, and how they will mould your future. Detailing the challenges of these difficult situations and how you dealt with them can be a useful asset to your personal statement. Think of situations like:

- Have you taken care of a family member?
- Has anyone in your family had an illness which affected you in any way?
- Have you been to the hospital or A&E for yourself or for your friends/family?
- Have you worked with people who have special needs?
- Have you spoken to a doctor or GP who has influenced you in any way?
- Has anyone you know suffered from pain?
- Have you seen a doctor treat in an empathetic way?
- Have you been impressed by the teamwork in your work experience?

If any of the above are relevant, think and reflect on how it has affected you. Then, try to write in a short sentence in your statement showing how this has influenced you to apply for medicine.

Awareness of the healthcare system

Some medical schools look for your awareness of the healthcare system and the nature of the medical training in your personal statement. It may be difficult to detail these within the space limit, but this will be extrapolated from your work experience and reflection.

Make it your own personal statement

Admissions staff look for statements that are personal rather than standard copied ones. Rather than stating 'I have always been interested in medicine and want to become a doctor', try to extrapolate from your personal experience and what motivated you to pursue medicine.

Common rules

Just like preparing for any document, it is vital:

- You get feedback from family members, advisers or teachers.
- Try writing, rewriting and revising it until you are happy with the version; start preparing early as this may need time.
- Use a spelling and grammar checker; silly mistakes and typos should be avoided.
- Check that this is a reflection of your work and volunteering experiences.
- Never use AI or ChatGPT to write; the admissions team can easily detect it. Your personal version is always preferred.

Structure of the statement

It should be well structured with an introduction and a conclusion. The introduction could be what motivated you to choose medicine. The conclusion could show your enthusiasm and curiosity. A few things to remember about the structure include:

- Make sure that it connects with the reader.
- Ensure there is a logical sequence to the structure of the statement.
- The statement should give confidence to the reader that you have done your research and are motivated to study medicine.
- The statement should be well constructed.
- Try to keep it concise and do not write unnecessary information; please do not repeat the same fact again anywhere in the statement.

Reflection is the key

The common mistake in many personal statements is that the candidate lists all the facts without reflecting on them. Even if you write three or four facts, if you have reflected well, that carries a higher value.

Give evidence for your statements. For example, do not just state that you are a conscientious person; give some evidence from your past experience. Do not just say that you know the value of empathy in medicine; give examples from your work experience or volunteering experience where you observed this.

Do not just stop by mentioning your extracurricular activities; reflect on how these skills can be transferred to medicine; or reflect on how this will help you towards your busy work as a doctor in the future.

Deadline for the personal statement

The deadline for a personal statement is when you submit the UCAS application; we suggest that you start working on it from the end of Year 12 or at least early during the summer break. This gives ample time for you to revise and rewrite it and to get advice from your teachers or career advisers.

Key Points

- UCAS is changing the personal statement format from one long piece to three separate texts from 2026.
- There will be a minimum 350-character count for each section, but the total character count for all three sections together will still be the same at 4000.
- Be honest and make it your own personal statement; avoid plagiarism.
- Personal life experiences can be valuable in showing what influenced you.
- Reflection is the key; just mentioning facts does not add value. Actively reflect on how this motivated you to do medicine.

References

1. UCAS. Medicine 2026 personal statement guide. Available from: https://www.ucas.com/applying/applying-university/writing-your-personal-statement/2026-personal-statement-guides/medicine-2026-personal-statement-guide.
2. UCAS. The new personal statement for 2026 entry. Available from: https://www.ucas.com/applying/applying-to-university/writing-your-personal-statement/the-new-personal-statement-for-2026.
3. University of Oxford. Medical Sciences Division. Medicine: anatomy of a personal statement. Available from: https://www.medsci.ox.ac.uk/study/medicine/pre-clinical/applying/anatomy-of-ps.

Chapter 11

Universities and Colleges Admissions Service (UCAS) application

In the United Kingdom, a candidate has to apply for universities through UCAS, which is an independent charity and is the UK's shared admissions service for higher education. The authors strongly recommend that students and parents familiarise themselves with the UCAS website (www.ucas.com) from the beginning of Year 12; however, UCAS can make changes and it is wise to keep continually looking for advice and guidelines on the website.

It is estimated that there are more than 23,000 applications for about 8000 medical school places (estimate from 2025 entry).

Please keep your UCAS ID number and login details safe as this will be needed to check and track the offers and if needed, to use the clearing system in the future.

Deadline for the UCAS application

The application system opens in September for a Year 13 candidate; this is the month when the school or college starts for Year 13. However, the entry courses will be shown on UCAS even from the end of April in Year 12 (for the following year entry).

A candidate has to submit an application online for courses in medicine on the UCAS website/portal by 18:00 hours UK time on the 15th October in their Year 13. This is much earlier than other undergraduate courses as there is a rigorous selection process followed by interviews in December to February for medicine. Your teacher should provide a reference in this application; your school will request you to submit the UCAS application to them a few days or weeks ahead of this final submission date; it is wise to liaise with the school and the career advice team. Please check with the UCAS website for application deadlines as they can change based on the university. It is not wise to wait until the last minute as the web system can get busy.

Application

A candidate needs to create an account on the UCAS web portal and fill out the online application form. Usually, the school or college will have sessions to help the candidate in this process. Once you fill in personal details, educational qualifications and work experience, you will need to submit a personal statement (see Chapter 10). You will then choose a maximum of four medical schools. You can use the fifth choice for a different course as a back-up, if you wish. Your UCAT results and scores will automatically be sent to the applied universities and you do not need to enter them. The standard course for medicine has a code of A100.

A UCAS medicine application costs £28.95 for the year 2026 but it may increase slightly and we advise checking with the UCAS website for the correct fees.

Reference

Your teacher will need time to prepare your reference and so the application needs to be submitted to them in advance of the UCAS submission deadline. Your teacher may not know what courses you are applying for on the UCAS website and so it is prudent to discuss your course and choices with them, so that they can write an appropriate reference. You will be giving only one reference for your application.

Tracking offers

Once a candidate completes interviews, offers start coming from December to April in Year 13 for medicine; this can vary between candidates and universities. This can be tracked through the UCAS system and usually the candidate also receives an email. For the fifth choice, which is a non-medicine course, the candidate might get an offer earlier.

Conditional offer

All medical schools only offer on condition that the candidate achieves the predicted grades or at least the minimum grade for selection that they mention on the offer. Usually this is AAA for most medical schools, but some ask for higher grades as there is huge competition, such as A*AA or A*A*A. We suggest that candidates prepare for a minimum of A*AA grades as competition becomes difficult every year.

The medical schools might also have conditions of health checks and vaccination checks as per the occupational health protocols.

Firm and insurance acceptance of offers

A candidate can receive a maximum of four offers from medical schools if they have done very well in all the stages. However, before the first week of June, they have to select two medical schools only and forfeit the others; out of these two, one of them will be a firm acceptance, which will be their first choice; the second one will be an insurance acceptance. As soon as you select this, the other two offers will be lost and given to others on the waiting list. In medicine, the insurance offer does not matter much, as the offer conditions are all similar to most medical schools except for a handful of schools that may want A*A*A or A*AA grades instead of AAA grades.

Application status on the UCAS platform

There are various statuses for your choices that can be marked on the UCAS platform, as follows:

1. Waiting for confirmation: it means that UCAS is waiting for the university to confirm if you have a place and have met the conditions.
2. Congratulations — choice offered: it means that you have got the place with a conditional offer; the conditions will be clear in the attached document, which is usually the grades achieved in the exams. You may get up to four offers depending on your performance in the interviews and the scores, but you should choose two of them in the time given on UCAS, which is usually the beginning of June. Within these two, you should choose a firm choice and an insurance choice.
3. You have not been placed at your choices: sorry, this means that you were not successful in your choices of medical schools; please check for the fifth option, which is not a medical school. If you have not been successful, you need to look for chances from the clearing system later on (explained in Chapter 16).
4. You have been offered a different course: if you do not get the A100 medicine course, the same university may offer you a different course (say, for example, a biomedical course, biological sciences, etc.). If you wish, you might take it, as it may need a lower grade or score compared with medicine; or you may wish to look at other options (discussed in Chapter 17).

Key Points

- The UCAS application deadline for medicine is 18:00 hours on the 15th October in Year 13.
- Please keep your UCAS ID number and login details safe; you will definitely need them in the future until you join the university.
- The candidate should start the application process early and give enough time for the teacher to submit their reference before the deadline.
- You can track offers on the UCAS website, but the candidate should also receive an email.
- All offers for medicine are conditional based on getting the minimum grades required for that medical school.
- A candidate should choose a firm and insurance offer at the beginning of June in Year 13.

References

1. UCAS. Applying. Available from: www.ucas.com/applying.
2. UCAS. What your application status means. Available from: https://www.ucas.com/applying/after-you-apply/clearing-and-results-day/results-day/what-your-application-status-means.

Chapter 12

Requirements for entry to medical schools

There are approximately 50 medical schools in the United Kingdom; the requirement criteria for entry into these schools vary slightly. Each candidate aspiring to be a doctor can only apply for four choices while filling in the UCAS application form; it is wise to choose these four options based on the candidate's particular strengths (see Chapter 13).

A candidate should already know what score they have achieved towards their requirement criteria while they apply to UCAS; they should know their GCSE scores, UCAT test scores, predicted A-level grades, etc. They should research the requirement criteria of each medical school and apply prudently. For example, it is not wise to apply to a university which gives a high value for UCAT scores if the candidate has not done well in the UCAT exam. This chapter will deal with the requirement criteria to enable the candidate to apply to the right place; these details are only correct at the time of publication of this book as taken from the website of each medical school/university. They can change regularly and we strongly advise the candidates and parents to check them before they apply. We have provided the website addresses for the universities/medical schools in this chapter.

University of Aberdeen — The School of Medicine, Medical Sciences and Nutrition

Website: https://www.abdn.ac.uk/smmsn/undergraduate/medicine/.

Applications are scored objectively by:

1. Academic achievements/predictions — 30%.
2. UCAT score — 20%.
3. Interview score — 50%.

To go to the interview stage, 60% academic prediction and 40% UCAT scores are required.

Minimum requirements:

- GCSEs: grade 6 in English Language and Mathematics with science subjects.
- SQA qualifications: five Highers at AAAB, A-levels with AAA (Chemistry is a must).
- UCAT score for the 2024 entry was an average of 2700 out of 3600 for those interviewed although there is no minimum cut-off.

Graduate entry is available. The multiple mini interview (MMI) format is used for interviews.

There is a virtual work experience available by students from the university; we recommend that candidates attend this if they want to apply to the Aberdeen School of Medicine.

Contact email: medadm@abdn.ac.uk.

Anglia Ruskin University School of Medicine

Website: https://www.aru.ac.uk/health-medicine-and-social-care/medicine.

Ranking for the interview is based on the UCAT score (after minimum academic entry requirements are checked).

Minimum requirements:

- GCSEs: five subjects at grade 6 minimum including English Language, Mathematics and two science subjects.
- A-levels: AAA with Chemistry or Biology.

The MMI format is used for interviews. There will be six interview stations, each lasting 7 minutes, with 1 minute to read the instructions between the stations. Candidates should be familiar with the NHS Constitution and the GMC requirements. Assessment will be made on interpersonal and communication skills (empathy), teamwork and leadership, preparation and motivation, critical thinking, ethical/moral reasoning, and integrity.

The Casper test was used in the 2023 admission although the scores were not taken into account.

Contact email: Admissions-SchoolofMedicine@aru.ac.uk.

Aston University Medical School, Birmingham

Website: https://www.aston.ac.uk/hls/aston-medical-school.

Total number of places: 110 for UK students and 30 places for international students.

Applications are ranked based on academic qualifications and the UCAT score. SJT banding is not considered.

Minimum requirements:

- GCSEs: six subjects at grade 6; must include English Language, Mathematics, Chemistry, Biology or Double Science.
- A-levels: A*AA with Chemistry and Biology compulsory.

The MMI format is used with specific assessments on understanding the study and practice of medicine with motivation, verbal communication, listening skills, teamwork, leadership skills, compassion, empathy, respect and dignity, and problem solving. The average score for those who received an offer in the entry year of 2024 was 50.1 out of 70. After the MMI interviews, candidates are re-ranked with the total score.

The UCAT score was an average of 2512 for applicants, 2722 for interviewees, and 2729 for those who received an offer in the 2024 entry year.

Contact email: ugadmissions@aston.ac.uk.

Bangor University, North Wales Medical School

Website: https://www.bangor.ac.uk/courses/undergraduate/a100-medicine-bmbs.

Minimum requirements:

- GCSEs: grade 6 in English Language, Double Science, Mathematics and four other subjects.
- A-levels: AAA, which include Biology and an additional science.

UCAT scores are used for ranking. The MMI format is used for interviews. Graduate entry is available.

Contact email: medicineadmissions@bangor.ac.uk.

University of Birmingham Medical School

Website: https://www.birmingham.ac.uk/schools/medical-school/applying-to-medicine/entry-requirements-five-year-programme.

Minimum requirements:

- GSCSEs: seven GCSEs will be scored for interview (English Language, Mathematics, Biology and Chemistry or Double Science — all at grade 6 minimum). Maximum score of 4 for grade 8/9 in the above-mentioned subjects, plus a score of 2 for grade 8/9 unspecified GCSE subjects. This total GCSE score is scaled to a maximum of 4.5.
- A-levels: A*AA including Biology and Chemistry. A-level scores at the first attempt are only taken into consideration.

UCAT scores: converted to scores based on the decile, with a maximum of 4 for scores above 2900. The SJT is not scored but is used at the interview stage.

The MMI format is used for interviews. Graduate entry is available. UCAT scores are needed.

Contact: fill in the enquiry form via their website at https://uob-admissions.powerappsportals.com/newenquiry/?source=MDS.

Brighton and Sussex Medical School

Website: https://www.bsms.ac.uk/undergraduate/applying-to-bsms/entry-requirements.aspx.

Minimum requirements:

- GCSEs: at least grade 6 in English (Language or Literature) and Mathematics.
- A-levels: AAA with Biology and Chemistry.

UCAT scores: used after assessing academic qualifications. SJT band score of 1, 2 or 3 only. UCAT minimum scores calculated for verbal reasoning, decision making and quantitative reasoning to give a total score of 2700 to rank the interview places.

The MMI format is used for interviews. Graduate entry is available.

Contact email: medamissions@bsms.ac.uk.

University of Bristol Medical School

Website address: https://www.bristol.ac.uk/medical-school/.

Minimum requirements:

- A-levels: AAA including Chemistry and either Biology, Physics, Mathematics or Further Mathematics.

A-levels and GCSEs are not weighted — they act as a cut-off.

The UCAT scores application is scored with 100% weighting on the UCAT result. There is no 'cut-off' score but the threshold for interview was 3010 for home applicants and 3080 for overseas applicants in 2025 (subject to change year on year).

Applicants are assessed using online MMI formats. Interview performance is ranked.

Graduate entry is available. UCAT scores are used for this pathway.

Contact email: medadmin-enquiries@bristol.ac.uk.

Brunel Medical School, Brunel University of London

Website: https://www.brunel.ac.uk/brunel-medical-school.

Minimum requirements:

- GCSEs: five subjects at grade 6/B including two science subjects (Double Science, Biology, Chemistry or Physics). Minimum of grade 4/C in English Language GCSE. Minimum of grade 5/B in Mathematics.
- A-levels: minimum of grades AAA–AAB; must include Chemistry or Biology at grade A, a second science (Chemistry, Biology, Physics) or Mathematics at grade A and a third subject (except General Studies) at grade A/B.

UCAT scores are used for ranking. SJT band 4 is excluded. Personal statements and references are assessed and satisfactory applicants will be ranked based on their UCAT scores.

A virtual (online) MMI format is used. Graduate entry is available; the Graduate Medical School Admissions Test (GAMSAT) is used for entry for graduates.

Contact email: BMS-Admissions@brunel.ac.uk.

University of Buckingham Medical School

Website: https://www.buckingham.ac.uk/medicine.

Minimum requirements:

- GCSEs: minimum of grade 4 in English and Mathematics.
- A-levels: minimum of grades ABB, including Chemistry and Biology.

UCAT scores are used for ranking. No admissions test is used.

Before the interview, candidates must attend a multiple mini assessment (MMA). This is a computer-based assessment similar to the SJT component of the UCAT.

The MMI format is used for interviews. Graduate entry is available with a minimum 2:1 Bachelor's degree in a field related to medicine.

Contact email: FMHS-admissions@buckingham.ac.uk.

University of Cambridge School of Clinical Medicine

Website: https://www.medschl.cam.ac.uk/.

Minimum requirements:

- A-levels: A*A*A including Chemistry and one other science or mathematics subject (Mathematics, Further Mathematics, Physics, Biology or Human Biology). Please consult their website as different colleges expect an A* in particular.

Graduate entry is available. A*A*A (or equivalent in other qualifications) if you graduated with a 2:1 or are yet to complete your degree. ABB (or equivalent in other qualifications) if you graduated with a first-class degree.

UCAT scores are used for ranking. The SJT score is not used. A panel interview format is used.

Contact email: admissions@cam.ac.uk.

Cardiff University School of Medicine

Website address: https://www.cardiff.ac.uk/medicine.

Minimum requirements:

- GCSEs: minimum of grade 6/B in English Language or Welsh Language. Grades 66/BB in GCSE Double Science or grade 6/B in Biology and

Chemistry separately. Grade 6/B in GCSE Mathematics. Five other GCSEs at a minimum grade of 6/B.
- A-levels: AAA; must include Biology and Chemistry.

UCAT scores: there is no cut-off score but ranking is used as the selection process.

The MMI format is used for interviews. Graduate entry is available. The applicant must have or be working towards a 2:1 honours degree and have BBB/ABC at A-level.

Contact email: medadmissions@cardiff.ac.uk.

City St George's University of London

Website: https://www.citystgeorges.ac.uk/prospective-students/subjects/medicine.

Minimum requirements:

- GCSEs: at least five subjects at grade 6/B and above; must include English Language, Mathematics, Science.
- A-levels: three A-level subjects.

UCAT scores are used for ranking. The SJT is included in the assessment criteria.

The MMI format is used for interviews. Asynchronous (video) interviews may be used in these stations. A graduate entry medicine programme is available.

Contact email: study@sgul.ac.uk.

University of Dundee School of Medicine

Website: https://www.dundee.ac.uk/medicine.

Minimum requirements:

- GCSEs: if not studied at A-level (A2), Biology or Chemistry at grade 7/A at GCSE.

- If not studied at A-level (A2), Mathematics and English at grade 6/B at GCSE.
- A-levels: AAA including Chemistry or Biology and another science (including Mathematics) (widening access ABB accepted).

UCAT scores are used for ranking.

The MMI format is used for interviews.

Contact email: medicine@dundee.ac.uk; asrs-medicine@dundee.ac.uk.

University of East Anglia, Norwich Medical School

Website: https://www.uea.ac.uk/course/undergraduate/mbbs-medicine.

Minimum requirements:

- GCSEs: minimum of six subjects at grade 7/A including Mathematics, Science, and grade 5/B in English Language.
- A-levels: AAA including Biology or Chemistry and two further subjects.

Two examples of relevant work experience are required.

UCAT scores are used to rank applicants, and the SJT score is added. UCAT (including SJT) and interview scores are added together for the final offer.

The MMI format is used for interviews. Graduate entry is available with a 2:1 class degree or above.

Contact email: admissions@uea.ac.uk or live chat available via https://www.uea.ac.uk/ask-us.

Edge Hill University Medical School

Website: https://www.edgehill.ac.uk/course/medicine/.

Minimum requirements:

- GCSEs: at least five subjects at grade 6/B or above including Biology, Chemistry, English Language and Mathematics.
- A-levels: AAA or A*AB with Biology and Chemistry.

The UCAT exam is needed. UCAT scores are used for invitation to the interviews. SJT band 4 is excluded.

The MMI format is used for interviews. Candidates are ranked as per MMI scores.

A graduate entry course and 6-year integrated version (with foundation year) are also available.

Contact email: askMedSchool@edgehill.ac.uk or online enquiry via https://www.edgehill.ac.uk/study/enquire/.

University of Edinburgh Medical School

Website: https://study.ed.ac.uk/programmes/undergraduate/354-mbchb-medicine-6-year-programme.
Website: https://medicine-vet-medicine.ed.ac.uk/edinburgh-medical-school/medicine/applying/how-to-apply/requirements.

This is a 6-year programme.

Minimum requirements:

- GCSEs: Biology at grade 7/A, Chemistry at grade 7/A, English at grade 7/A, Mathematics at grade 7/A.
- A-levels: A*AA; required to take Chemistry, and one from Biology, Human Biology, Mathematics/Further Mathematics or Physics.

UCAT scores are used for ranking. The 2026 entry cut-off score is 1650. If the cut-off is met, scores are ranked into deciles. SJT band 3 or higher only. Points from the SJT and UCAT overall scores are added to the academic score and contribute to the final ranking.

The interview is in an assessment-day format; this is a half-day assessment with a series of short interviews.

Personal statements are used to guide assessment days and should be prepared before the interview.

Contact email: mbchbcoordinator@ed.ac.uk.

University of Exeter Medical School

Website: https://medicine.exeter.ac.uk/.
Website: https://www.exeter.ac.uk/study/undergraduate/courses/medicine/medicine/.

Minimum requirements:

- GCSEs: grade 6/B in English Language.
- A-levels: A*AA with Chemistry and Biology.

UCAT scores are used for ranking.

Graduate entry is available; the GAMSAT test is used for ranking. The MMI format is used for interviews.

Contact: enquiry online via https://www.exeter.ac.uk/about/enquiry/.

University of Glasgow Medical School

Website: https://www.gla.ac.uk/undergraduate/degrees/medicine/#/entryrequirements,entryrequirements.

Minimum requirements:

- GCSEs: Biology and English Language or Literature at grade 6/B.
- A-levels: AAA, Chemistry compulsory, one of either Biology, Physics or Mathematics.

UCAT scores are used for ranking.

Interviews — a panel interview online via Zoom; two interviewers covering both panel and B.

Graduate entry is available with a minimum 2:1 honours degree in science; the UCAT scores are used for ranking.

Contact email: med-sch-admissions@glasgow.ac.uk.

Hull York Medical School

Website: https://www.hyms.ac.uk/medicine/mbbs-medicine.

Minimum requirements:

- GCSEs: six subjects at grade 6/B or above in English Language and Mathematics.
- A-levels: AAB with Biology and Chemistry.

UCAT scores are used for ranking. SJT band 4 is excluded.

The MMI format is used for interviews. Various sections are used including group exercise (22 points), two mini interviews (2 × 17 points), a student station run by medical students (17 points), an individual scenario station with a pre-recorded video simulation (17 points). The online interview has a different scoring system.

Contact email: admissions@hyms.ac.uk.

Imperial College London School of Medicine

Website: https://www.imperial.ac.uk/study/courses/undergraduate/medicine/.

This is a 6-year course with an intercalated BSc.

Minimum requirements:

- A-levels: AAA to include Biology and Chemistry.

UCAT scores are used to rank for invitations to the interviews. SJT band 4 is excluded.

The minimum threshold for UCAT is approximately 2122 for the new entry (it was 2830 in the old system).

The MMI format is used for interviews.

Contact email: medicine.ug.admissions@imperial.ac.uk.

Keele University School of Medicine

Website address: https://www.keele.ac.uk/medicine/.

Minimum requirements:

- GCSEs: five subjects at grade 7/A, with a minimum of grade 6/B in English Language, Mathematics, Biology, Chemistry and Physics.
- A-levels: A*AA or AAA+EPQ grade A, Biology or Chemistry is compulsory as the first subject.

The personal statement is scored along with the UCAT score for a total on a scale of 1–25. If scores are the same for two candidates, the UCAT verbal reasoning score is taken to decide on the best candidate. Please note observership is not counted in the personal statement and see the school's website on the personal statement before submitting to UCAS at: https://www.keele.ac.uk/media/k-web/k-study/coursepages/undergraduate/Guidance%20notes%20for%20Keele%20medicine%20personal%20statement%202026.pdf.

UCAT scores are a minimum of 1700. SJT band 4 is excluded.

Graduate entry is available; need to take both GAMSAT and UCAT.

Interviews are conducted online using Microsoft Teams. Two 15-minute interviews, usually 2 hours apart, are the format; candidates are required to read some materials that will be provided in advance (usually 1–2 days before).

Contact email: medicine@keele.ac.uk.

Kent and Medway Medical School

Website: https://kmms.ac.uk/entry-requirements-2026/.

Minimum requirements:

- GCSEs: five subjects at grade 6/B minimum; must include English Language, Mathematics, Biology, Chemistry and Physics (or Double Science and one other subject).
- A-levels: AAB, Chemistry and/or Biology; if not, then one from Physics, Mathematics, Psychology or Computer Science allowed.

Does not use predicted grades; uses only achieved grades for selection.

UCAT scores: threshold corresponding to the 47th centile accepted (2490 in the old system), and SJT 3 or above. These thresholds may vary next year.

In stage 2b, applicants are contextualised relative to their school average; absolute grade attainments are not used but only relative attainment based on schooling. The school states that the interview preparation courses may be less useful as they try to find the true version of the candidate.

The MMI format is used for interviews. Graduate entry is available.

Contact email: admissions@kmms.ac.uk.

King's College London GKT School of Medical Education

Website: https://www.kcl.ac.uk/study/undergraduate/courses/medicine-mbbs.

Minimum requirements:

- GCSEs: grade 6/B minimum in English Language and Mathematics.
- A-levels: A*AA, Chemistry and Biology required; EPQ is not considered.

UCAT scores: there is no threshold; the overall score including the SJT is taken into account when shortlisting.

A personal statement is also considered before an interview. Interviews are held. An online MMI format is used.

Contact: telephone number +44 020 7836 5454.

Lancaster Medical School

Website: https://www.lancaster.ac.uk/study/undergraduate/courses/medicine-and-surgery-mbchb-a100/2025/.

Minimum requirements:

- GCSEs: minimum score of 13 points from eight subjects (grade 6/B is 1 point, while grades 7–9/A or A* is 2 points); if Biology or Chemistry is not studied at A-level, GCSE must be at least grade 7/A.
- A-levels: AAA with any two of Biology, Chemistry and Psychology; AAB accepted with a B in a fourth subject or EPQ.

UCAT scores are used for ranking.

The MMI format is used for interviews.

Contact email: medicine@lancaster.ac.uk.

University of Leeds School of Medicine

Website: https://courses.leeds.ac.uk/5580/medicine-and-surgery-mbchb.

Minimum requirements:

- GCSEs: minimum of six subjects including Mathematics, English Language, Biology and Chemistry or Double Science. Scoring is actually based on eight GCSEs while shortlisting.
- A-levels: AAA including Chemistry and Biology. No advantage in taking a fourth subject as A* and A are treated the same. EPQs are not considered.

UCAT scores are used for ranking.

The MMI format is used for interviews.

Contact email: ugmadmissions@leeds.ac.uk.

Leicester Medical School

Website: https://le.ac.uk/courses/medicine-mbchb/2026.

Minimum requirements:

- GCSEs: at least grade 6/B in English Language, Mathematics, and two sciences. GCSE grades scored for 50% from eight subjects for pre-interview selection.
- A-levels: A*AA, includes Chemistry or Biology, and one of Biology, Chemistry, Physics, Mathematics or Psychology, and a third subject. AAA grades are considered with an EPQ or AAAB (two science subjects at A).

UCAT scores: form 50% of the pre-interview scoring system. SJT band 4 is excluded.

The MMI format is used for interviews. Graduate entry is available.

Contact email: medadmis@le.ac.uk.

Lincoln Medical School

Website: https://www.lincoln.ac.uk/course/mdcmbcub/.

Minimum requirements:

- GCSEs: at least six subjects at grade 7 or above; must include Biology, Chemistry or Double Science. Grade 6 minimum required in English Language and Mathematics.
- A-levels: AAA; must include Biology.

UCAT scores are used for ranking. SJT band 4 is excluded.

The MMI format is used for interviews.

Contact email: enquiries@lincoln.ac.uk.

University of Liverpool School of Medicine

Website: https://www.liverpool.ac.uk/medicine/.

Minimum requirements:

- GCSEs: at least five subjects at grade 6/B; must include English Language, Mathematics and Science.
- A-levels: AAA; must include Chemistry, a second subject of either Biology, Physics or Mathematics, and a third subject. A*AB accepted if A* in Chemistry, A in Biology, Physics or Mathematics, and B in the third subject.

UCAT scores and the SJT are used for selection for interviews.

The MMI format is used for interviews. Graduate entry is available; the GAMSAT test is essential. Minimum of a 2:1 honours degree in any subject.

Contact email: mbchb@liverpool.ac.uk.

University of Manchester School of Medical Sciences

Website: https://www.manchester.ac.uk/study/undergraduate/courses/2026/01428/mbchb-medicine/.

Manchester has 401 funded places for medicine and has one of the largest numbers of medical school places.

Minimum requirements:

- GCSEs: minimum of seven subjects at grade 7/A or above, with English Language, Mathematics, and at least two science subjects at a minimum of grade 6/B.

- A-levels: AAA including Biology or Chemistry, second subject of Chemistry, Biology, Physics, Psychology, Mathematics or Further Mathematics.

UCAT scores are used for ranking. SJT band 1 or 2 only is included.

The MMI format is used for interviews, either online via Zoom or in person. Graduate entry is available.

Contact email: ug.medicine@manchester.ac.uk.

University of Greater Manchester Medical School, Bolton

Website: https://greatermanchester.ac.uk/course/mbchb-medicine-full-time-5-years-university-of-bolton.

This is a new medical school, accepting only international applicants for 2025.

Minimum requirements:

- GCSEs: minimum of five subjects at grade 6 or above; must include Mathematics, English Language, and two sciences.
- A-levels: AAB, including Chemistry or Biology, second subject of Biology, Chemistry, Physics or Mathematics, and a third subject.

The personal statement is assessed during shortlisting for interviews.

UCAT scores are used for ranking.

Online MMIs are used with tests. Graduate entry is available with a 2:1 honours degree from any discipline.

Contact email: mbchbadmissions@bolton.ac.uk.

Newcastle University Medical School

Website: https://www.ncl.ac.uk/undergraduate/degrees/a100/.

Minimum requirements:

- GCSEs: best eight subjects considered. This will be converted to academic grades with a score out of 40.
- A-levels: AAA in any subject.

UCAT scores are used for ranking. This will be converted to a maximum of 60 points. SJT band 4 is excluded.

The MMI format is used for interviews. The final score is based on the academic screen score and interview score, weighted 50:50.

Contact email: mbbs.admissions@ncl.ac.uk.

University of Nottingham School of Medicine

Website: https://www.nottingham.ac.uk/studywithus/ugstudy/courses/UG/Medicine-BMBS-U6UBMBSC3.html.

Minimum requirements:

- GCSEs: minimum of six subjects at grade 7/A, including Biology and Chemistry.
- A-levels: AAA; must include Biology and Chemistry.

UCAT scores are used for ranking. GCSE and UCAT scores are used to short-list for interviews. The SJT is included in the assessment criteria, but SJT band 4 is excluded; usually, due to competition, only SJT band 1 will be offered interviews. If GCSE not taken, the UCAT scores are used alone.

Online MMI interviews using Microsoft Teams are used; six scenarios, including at least one role-play station. Graduate entry is available.

Contact: online form at https://enquiry-form.powerappsportals.com/get-intouch/?referrer=https://www.nottingham.ac.uk/help-and-support/home/contact-us.html.

University of Oxford Medical School

Website: https://www.ox.ac.uk/admissions/undergraduate/courses/course-listing/medicine.

This is a 6-year course.

Minimum requirements:

- A-levels: A*AA with Chemistry and at least one of Biology, Physics, Mathematics or Further Mathematics, and a third subject.

Two college choices; one chosen by the candidate and one randomly allocated.

UCAT scores are used for ranking.

Online panel interviews are used.

There is no separate pathway for graduates, but they can apply for the standard course.

Contact email: admissions@medschool.ox.ac.uk.

University of Plymouth (Peninsula Medical School)

Website: https://www.plymouth.ac.uk/courses/undergraduate/bmbs-bachelor-of-medicine-bachelor-of-surgery.

Minimum requirements:

- GCSEs: minimum of seven subjects at a minimum grade 4/C, which includes English Language, Mathematics and two science subjects.
- A-levels: AAA with Biology, second subject of Chemistry, Physics, Mathematics or Psychology, and a third subject.

UCAT scores and GCSEs are used to shortlist for interviews.

An online MMI format is used for interviews. Graduate entry is available; GAMSAT is used for the assessment.

Contact email: admissions@plymouth.ac.uk; meddent-admissions@plymouth.ac.uk.

University of Central Lancashire School of Medicine & Dentistry, Preston

Website: https://www.lancashire.ac.uk/undergraduate/courses/medicine-mbbs.

UCLAN has more international student places, and only 50 places for UK students.

Minimum requirements:

- GCSEs: Mathematics and English at grade 5/B.
- A-levels: AAA with at least two science subjects including Chemistry.

UCAT scores are used for ranking.

The MMI format is used for interviews. Graduate entry is available with a 2:1 honours degree in science or health.

Contact email: ia@uclan.ac.uk.

Queen Mary University of London, Barts and The London School of Medicine and Dentistry

Website: https://www.qmul.ac.uk/undergraduate/coursefinder/courses/2025/medicine-5-year-programme/.

Minimum requirements:

- GCSEs: six subjects with grades 777666/AAABB including Biology, Chemistry, English Language or Literature, and Mathematics.
- A-levels: A*AA; must include Biology or Chemistry, second subject of Chemistry or Biology or Physics or Mathematics, and a third subject.

UCAT scores with fourth decile or above. SJT bands 1–3.

Panel interviews are used, online at present.

Graduate entry is available with a 2:1 class degree in any subject with supporting Biology and Chemistry qualifications.

Contact email: smdadmissions@qmul.ac.uk.

Queen's University Belfast School of Medicine

Website: https://www.qub.ac.uk/courses/undergraduate/medicine-mb-a100/.

Minimum requirements:

- GCSEs: grade 4/C minimum in Mathematics, Physics or Double Science. GCSEs in the best nine subjects will be scored with points according to their grades.
- A-levels: A*AA or AAAA, should include Chemistry and another subject from Biology, Mathematics or Physics; Biology essential at AS-level at least. AAA with EPQ grade A is also considered.

UCAT scores are used for ranking. UCAT and GCSEs scores will be added to rank candidates for interviews.

The MMI format is used for interviews. Graduate applicants are scored with UCAT. Minimum 2:1 honours grade in their first undergraduate degree, which can be from a wide range of different subjects.

Contact email: admissions.med@qub.ac.uk; admissions@qub.ac.uk.

University of Sheffield School of Medicine

Website: https://sheffield.ac.uk/smph/undergraduate/medicine-admissions.

Minimum requirements:

- GCSEs: five subjects at grade 7/A with at least grade 6/B in Mathematics, English Language and the science subjects.

- A-levels: AAA with Chemistry or Biology, a second science subject, and a third subject; or AAB with an A in the EPQ.

UCAT scores: minimum threshold of 1800/2700 for 2026 entry.

The MMI format is used for interviews; a knowledge of Sheffield will be tested in one station. MMI and SJT scores are added together for a total score of 45. Graduate entry is available with a 1:1 class Bachelor's degree with BBB at A-level.

Contact email: medadmissions@sheffield.ac.uk.

University of Southampton School of Medicine

Website: https://www.southampton.ac.uk/study/subjects/medicine.

Minimum requirements:

- GCSEs: minimum of seven subjects at grade 6/B; should include English Language, Mathematics and Science.
- A-levels: AAA to include Biology and one additional science (Chemistry, Physics, Psychology, Sociology, Environmental studies or Geography).

UCAT scores are used for ranking.

Selection days consist of traditional panel interviews and group exercises.

Contact email: AdmissionsUG.MED@southampton.ac.uk.

University of St Andrews School of Medicine

Website: https://www.st-andrews.ac.uk/medicine/.

This is a 6-year course. Students graduate with a BSc (Hons) Medicine from St Andrews and then progress to partner medical schools after 3 years to complete an MBChB or MBBS.

Minimum requirements:

- GCSEs: minimum of five subjects at grade 7/A.
- A-levels: AAA including Chemistry and one of Biology, Mathematics or Physics. If Biology is not taken, the candidate should have achieved grade 5/B in GCSEs.

Personal statements, relevant medically related work experience, and a positive reference are used to shortlist for interviews.

UCAT scores are used for ranking.

The MMI format is used for interviews; four mini-interview stations are held. Graduate entry is available with an upper second or first class honours degree in science.

Contact email: medical.admissions@st-andrews.ac.uk.

St Mary's School of Medicine, Twickenham

Website: https://www.stmarys.ac.uk/courses/undergraduate/mbbs-medicine-degree.

This school opens in 2026; it only accepts international students.

Minimum requirements:

- GCSEs: minimum of grade 6 in Mathematics, English Language, Biology and Chemistry or Double Science.
- A-levels: AAA with Chemistry or Biology, second subject in science (Biology, Chemistry, Physics or Mathematics), and a third subject.

UCAT scores are used for ranking.

The MMI format is used for interviews.

Contact email: apply@stmarys.ac.uk.

University of Sunderland School of Medicine

Website: https://www.sunderland.ac.uk/study/medicine/mbchb-medicine/.

Minimum requirements:

- GCSEs: five subjects at grade 7/A; minimum of grade 6 in Mathematics, English Language, Biology, Chemistry and Physics.
- A-levels: AAA; must include Biology or Chemistry, and a second subject in science (Biology, Chemistry, Physics, Mathematics/Further Mathematics/Statistics), and a third subject.

UCAT scores are needed, top 8 deciles of cohort, with SJT in bands 1–3 only.

The MMI format is used for interviews. Graduate entry is available; 5-year standard course; 2:1 in any subject with BBB in A-levels needed.

Contact email: medicineapplications@sunderland.ac.uk; student.helpline@sunderland.ac.uk.

Swansea University Medical School

Website: https://www.swansea.ac.uk/undergraduate/courses/medicine/medicine-graduate-entry-mbbch/.

Only graduate entry medicine course available in Swansea (A101 UCAS code); cannot be chosen after A-levels. Total of 150 spaces available for graduate entry.

Minimum requirements:

- Minimum grade C at GCSE in Maths and English/Welsh.
- Minimum 2:1 honours degree in undergraduate course in any subject, or Merit in an integrated master's degree, or 2:2 honours undergraduate degree and a pass in a postgraduate higher degree in any subject.

GAMSAT or UCAT test is needed.

Assessments will consist of 3 x 20–30 minute face-to-face stations in the form of questions/discussions, presentations or role-play scenarios. The personal statement may be questioned in one of these stations. The interview is structured to take account of the qualities needed as a doctor, as set out in the GMC's *Good Medical Practice*; the interview tests communication skills, problem-solving skills, coping with pressure, insight and integrity, passion for medicine and resilience, organisation and research, and ethics/values.

Contact email: admissions@swansea.ac.uk.

University College London Medical School

Website: https://www.ucl.ac.uk/prospective-students/undergraduate/degrees/medicine-mbbs-bsc.

This is a 6-year programme.

Minimum requirements:

- GCSEs: minimum of grade 6/B in English Language and Mathematics.
- A-levels: A*AA with Biology and Chemistry.

UCAT scores are used for ranking; when scores are similar, SJT scores are used to further rank each candidate.

The MMI format is used for interviews.

Contact: telephone +44 20 8059 0939 or via the online form at https://www.ucl.ac.uk/prospective-students/undergraduate/admissions-enquiries.

University of Warwick Medical School

Website: https://warwick.ac.uk/fac/sci/med/.

This is only a graduate entry medicine course (A101 UCAS code) available in Warwick. There are a total of 193 places available every year.

Minimum requirements:

- Upper second class honours (2:1) degree in any subject; or lower second class with Master's or doctoral qualification.

UCAT is essential.

At least 70 hours of health- or social care-related work experience in the last 3 years is needed; these should be in at least two different health or social care organisations and at least two roles/professions.

The MMI format is used for interviews

Contact email: mbchb.admissions@warwick.ac.uk.

Other universities/medical schools

This chapter has not covered several universities including:

- University of Surrey Medical School — started 2025. A graduate entry course.
- Ulster University — only graduate entry courses; uses GAMSAT for assessment.
- Pears Cumbria School of Medicine, Carlisle — starts from 2026. Only graduate entry courses; uses UCAT or GAMSAT for assessment.
- University of Chester School of Medicine — plans for the future.
- Three Counties Medical School, Worcester — plans for the future.

Research before applying

It is prudent to carry out extensive research before applying on the UCAS forms. The suggestions we have given are based on medical school websites for 2026 and they change every year. Please make sure you check the recent recommendations well in advance and analyse the information properly before applying.

You should carefully consider your academic achievements and your personal situation before applying. There is some flexibility as each medical school differs to some extent in their basic entry requirements. For example, if you have not taken Biology at A-level, you could still apply if you have the complementary subjects as mentioned in the entry requirements of those medical schools. Some examples of such schools include Aberdeen, Anglia Ruskin, Bristol, Brunel, Cambridge, Dundee, East Anglia, Edinburgh, Glasgow and Keele. You could also research the requirements without Biology in various medical schools such as Birmingham, Leicester, Liverpool, Manchester, Newcastle, Oxford, Plymouth, Queen Mary, Sheffield, St Andrews and Sunderland. Lancaster may also consider skipping Biology if you have Psychology. Please check the medical school websites as the chances of getting an interview may vary despite these allowances.

If you drop a grade in A-levels, then having a B grade or more in an EPQ may help in some medical schools such as Lancaster, Leicester and Sheffield. An EPQ is not used in some schools such as Birmingham, King's College London and Plymouth. Again, please check their websites before deciding on the choice of subjects.

If you have a fourth A-level subject, it may add to the pressure in exam preparation but some schools may consider a B grade in a 4th subject to reduce the grade in one of the other three subjects; for example, Leicester may accept a grade of AAAB instead of A*AA. Please check the website again before selecting the subject.

If your English score is reduced in the GCSE, there may still be possibilities for medical schools such as Bristol, Brunel, East Anglia and Plymouth. If your GCSE scores are reduced, you might consider Cambridge, Oxford, Buckingham or Imperial Collge as they look at other criteria. If you only achieve AAB grades rather than AAA grades at A-level, consider Hull, or you could consider Lancaster if you achieve a grade B in a fourth subject or in an EPQ. If your UCAT score is low, some universities may be generous in offering interviews such as Kent and Medway. If your predicted grade is less, you may still get an interview for Kent and Medway. These are predictions that may change in the future and we strongly advise you to conduct thorough research and check the most recent entry criteria from the websites of medical schools.

The requirements for entry to medical schools is shown in ■ Table 12.1.

Table 12.1. Requirements for entry to medical schools.

	University	GCSE	A-levels	UCAT	SJT	Interview	Number of applicants per place	Number of applicants per interview
1	Aberdeen	30%		20%		MMI — 50%	6	2
2	Anglia Ruskin	Minimum	AAA	100%		MMI	15	3
3	Aston	24	A*AA	Ranked	Not scored	MMI		
4	Bangor		AAA	Ranked		MMI		
5	Birmingham	4.5	A*AA	4.0	Interview	MMI	6.6	2.2
6	Brighton Sussex	Minimum	AAA	Ranked	1, 2, 3	MMI		
7	Bristol	Minimum	AAA	100%		Online MMI		
8	Brunel	Minimum	AAA or AAB	Ranked	1, 2, 3	Online MMI		
9	Buckingham	Minimum	ABB	UCAT and MMA		MMI		
10	Cambridge	Minimum	A*A*A	Ranked	Not used	Panel		
11	Cardiff	Minimum	AAA	Ranked		MMI		
12	City St George	Minimum		Ranked	Included	MMI	8	2
13	Dundee	Minimum	AAA	Ranked		MMI		
14	East Anglia, Norwich	Minimum	AAA	Ranked	Included final score	MMI		
15	Edge Hill	Minimum	AAA or A*AB	Ranked	1, 2, 3	MMI		
16	Edinburgh	Minimum	A*AA	Ranked	1, 2, 3	Assessment day	7	3
17	Exeter	Minimum	A*AA	Ranked		MMI	7	2
18	Glasgow	Minimum	AAA	Ranked		Panel		
19	Hull	Minimum	AAB	Ranked	1, 2, 3	MMI	8	2

Continued overleaf

Table 12.1. Requirements for entry to medical schools.

	University	GCSE	A-levels	UCAT	SJT	Interview	Number of applicants per place	Number of applicants per interview
20	Imperial College London	Minimum	AAA	Ranked	1, 2, 3	MMI	10	3
21	Keele	Minimum	A*AA or AAA+EPQ	Ranked	1, 2, 3	Online panel	16	4
22	Kent and Medway	Minimum	AAB	Minimum score only	1, 2, 3	MMI	18	4
23	King's College London	Minimum	A*AA	Ranked No threshold		Online MMI	10	4
24	Lancaster	Points 13 out of 16	AAA or AABB or AAB with EPQ	Ranked		MMI	7.8	2.2
25	Leeds	Minimum but 8 subjects scored	AAA	Ranked		MMI	7	2.5
26	Leicester	Scored for 50%	A*AA or AAAB or AAB with EPQ	Scored for 50%	1, 2, 3	MMI	8	2
27	Lincoln	Minimum	AAA	Ranked	1, 2, 3	MMI		
28	Liverpool	Minimum	AAA or A*AB	Ranked	Interview	MMI	8.9	1.4
29	Manchester	Minimum	AAA	Ranked	1, 2	MMI	2	1.5
30	University of Greater Manchester	Minimum	AAB; only inter-national students	Ranked		MMI and tests		

Continued overleaf

Table 12.1. Requirements for entry to medical schools.

	University	GCSE	A-levels	UCAT	SJT	Interview	Number of applicants per place	Number of applicants per interview
31	Newcastle	Minimum academic score	AAA	Ranked	1, 2, 3	MMI	6	2.5
32	Nottingham	Minimum	AAA	Ranked	1, 2, 3	Online MMI	10	3
33	Oxford	Minimum	A*AA	Ranked		Online panel	10	2.5
34	Plymouth	Minimum	AAA	Ranked		Online MMI		
35	University of Central Lancashire, Preston	Minimum	AAA	Ranked		MMI		
36	Queen Mary London	Minimum	A*AA	Ranked	1, 2, 3	Online panel	5.8	1.8
37	Queen's Belfast	Minimum	A*AA or AAAA or AAA with EPQ grade A	Ranked		MMI		
38	Sheffield	Minimum	AAA or AAB with A in EPQ	Ranked	Added to final score	MMI	7	3.8
39	Southampton	Minimum	AAA	Ranked		Panel and group exercise		
40	St Andrews	Minimum	AAA	Ranked		MMI	10	3
41	St Mary's Twickenham	Minimum	AAA	Ranked		MMI		

Continued overleaf

Table 12.1. Requirements for entry to medical schools.

	University	GCSE	A-levels	UCAT	SJT	Interview	Number of applicants per place	Number of applicants per intervie[w]
42	Sunderland	Minimum	AAA	Ranked	1, 2, 3	MMI	10	2.4
43	Swansea (graduate entry)	C in Maths, English	Not used	GAMSAT or UCAT		Assessment panel	5	1.5
44	University College London	Minimum	A*AA	Ranked	Used to rank	MMI	7	2
45	Warwick (graduate entry)			Ranked		MMI		

Key Points

- **All medical schools have specific entry criteria.**
- **These can change in the next academic year.**
- **It is best to check the website regularly and see the requirements for the year of your admission.**

References

1. Medical Schools Council. UK medical school entry requirements. Available from: https://www.medschools.ac.uk/for-students/applying-to-medical-school/entry-requirements/?course_type=standard-entry-medicine.

Chapter 13

How to select the right medical school

It is a difficult task for a candidate to select just four choices of medical schools when applying to the UCAS system from nearly 50 medical schools in the UK. Some students may have a particular liking for the city where the medical school is located and they want to spend their next 5–6 years in that city. Some want to go to a medical school where the hospital and facilities are reputable. Some want to go to a big city where the university has a good reputation. However, for medicine, most of the courses have the same outcome when managing the guidelines set by the GMC.

When a candidate finishes 5 years of medical school, they have to apply on an online system for the 2-year foundation year programme; at this stage, the candidate may also be allocated to a totally different geographical area.

The aim of this chapter is to provide guidance on how to get the best results in the selection process from the existing academic and other achievements of the candidate. For selecting the facilities and curriculum, the candidate should attend open days at the universities (see Chapter 7) and visit the websites of the various medical schools to research the available structure and outcomes (see Chapter 12).

City and the location

For most students, the location of the medical school may be an important criterion for choosing it. It may be the city or the campus that attracts a candidate, but they are going to spend the next 5–6 years there and it is vital that this is a key selection which is researched well. A candidate may place importance upon various facilities including the accommodation, facilities available, and travel possibilities to hospitals and clinical placements.

Teaching styles in the medical school

Medical schools can differ in the way teaching is delivered; it is vital to look at their website and research this before you apply. Traditional teaching is delivered in the classroom in the first 2 years and then moves to a clinical setting in the third year; very few schools have this approach now.

Integrated teaching combines both the classroom and the clinical setting teaching right from the start; the curriculum is based on systems rather than by a subject.

Problem-based teaching gives a real-life problem, which is researched by the student, who will then acquire new skills and knowledge through a self-directed learning approach.

Enquiry-based teaching is question-driven and is also student self-centred; the student investigates the questions, explores ideas and constructs their own understanding.

Each candidate may have their own preference in which they flourish in a particular teaching environment; some may be open to all techniques.

Entry requirements criteria

This is the area where many students need to concentrate; unless you read the requirements (see Chapter 12) for each medical school and analyse if you can score well to get into that school, it will be a waste of a choice. The authors recommend shortlisting 6–8 universities, then going to their website and looking at all the criteria; these are the essential minimums needed for entry to that medical school. The next step would be to find out what the cut-off was for the previous year and see if you will fit into the criteria; there could be slight changes for this year, but it is wise to predict and analyse these cut-off scores.

Some medical schools place huge importance on GCSE scores while selecting candidates for the interviews. If you have scored well at GCSE level, this is a bonus point for you; if not, then you should avoid choosing these medical schools and look at other options.

Some schools place higher importance on UCAT scores; some place importance on SJT banding. Please research what was the cut-off for the previous year. For example, some medical schools had listed in the entry criteria that a SJT band of 1, 2, 3 was needed and only band 4 was eliminated, but then on checking who was selected in the previous year, only SJT band 1 were selected for interview and many candidates did not realise this and wasted a choice in the UCAS system (despite having great predicted A-level grades and a very high total UCAT score). The minimum criterion does not mean that you will be selected for the interview as the competition increases every year; so, it is vital that you check the previous year's selection cut-off.

As you would have shortlisted 6–8 medical schools, it is prudent to do your research and look at the criteria and last year's success cut-offs in detail before choosing the four choices in the UCAS application.

Academic achievements and subjects

Medical schools vary in their requirement of subjects learnt at both GCSE and A-levels; do some research as you can easily find the medical school to fit your own criteria. For example, if you have not done Biology at A-level, you can still select a few medical schools that accept without Biology. See Chapter 12 and the medical school's website for the particular details, as these can also vary and change in the future.

If you have studied Chemistry and Biology, the options increase when choosing medical schools.

Personal statement and work experience

Most medical schools do not select based on the personal statement while a few do. Most schools do not score on work experience (but expect you to mention it at the MMI station), but some like Warwick (graduate entry) may ask for a document to be filled in, which will be scored. Some do not accept observership but want work experience, even if it is in a related field.

How competitive is medical school?

It is also important to find out the competition ratios, both for application and success rates in the interviews; most medical schools have the data (see Table 12.1) but check the recent data. If a medical school is asking for A*AA instead of AAA, it means that it may be more competitive. It may be worth looking at the total number of places available in that university to study medicine. If you are particular about applying for a course that has high competition, make sure that you choose an easier one for the third and fourth choices as a back-up. Similarly, you can choose a medical school asking for A*AA as your first choice, but have a school with AAA or AAB as one of the choices if your grade falls in the exams.

Cost of living

The financial burden is significant for a student in medical school; the student pays the tuition fees, but there are additional living expenses that should be calculated. Living in a big city will cost more compared with living in a rural area; however, this may depend on the preference of the candidate.

Integrated degrees

Some universities offer intercalated or integrated courses and offer a BSc or MSc qualification along with the medical degree. The downside is that the candidate will be spending one extra year at school, while the benefits include exposure to research and innovation. Depending on the medical school, this could be optional or compulsory.

It is estimated that nearly 23,000 candidates apply for the 8000 medical school places in the UK. It is extremely competitive. Many of the candidates fail in this process because they have not applied to the right medical school where their academic achievements and other scores will fit the entry requirements. It is worth spending time researching where you will fit the criteria for entry.

Key Points

- **From nearly 50 medical schools in the UK, a candidate can only choose to apply for four. It is vital to do the research and choose them wisely.**
- **The candidate should check that they fit the entry requirements, but also see what was the cut-off for selection in the previous year.**
- **Attending open days may help to make the decision; a candidate will be spending the next 5–6 years in the city and it is vital to make sure that they like the city and the campus.**

References

1. British Medical Association. Applying to medical school. Nov 2024. Available from: https://www.bma.org.uk/advice-and-support/studying-medicine/becoming-a-doctor/applying-to-medical-school.
2. Medical Schools Council. Medical Schools A-Z. Available from: https://www.medschools.ac.uk/for-students/applying-to-medical-school/medical-schools/.

Chapter 14

Interviews for the medical school

Medical schools use interviews as one of the assessment tools to select the right candidate for the career. Most of the schools have moved towards the multiple mini interview (MMI) station format as this has an organised structure and avoids bias. A very small number of schools still have panel interviews. The basis of both interviews is the same: to select the right candidate who has motivation, has done some research about the medical school, has some work experience, understands the ethics of medicine, and has knowledge of the pros and cons of the career. A medical career can be stressful and it is essential that medical schools select the right candidate to avoid them leaving the profession or course later.

This chapter can only give a summary of the process of the interview but, for better preparation for the interviews, the authors recommend the book: *Interviews for Medical School: Multiple Mini Interview (MMI) Practice*, ISBN 978-1-913755-32-4, published by the same publisher (tfm publishing Ltd). This book has received excellent feedback and the royalties from the sales of the book go fully to charitable causes via a charity.

Selection of interviews

Once the UCAS application has been submitted in October in Year 13, the universities have a chance to shortlist the candidates for interviews. Each medical school has their own way of selecting the candidates for these interviews and these criteria are clearly evident on their website; see Chapter 12 for more details on requirements for medical school, but check their website for recent changes or updates in these criteria. It is wise to achieve good grades in GCSEs and good UCAT scores to have a high probability of being selected for the interviews. However, the minimum predicted grade for A-levels (as submitted by the school based on Year 12 performances) will be checked before the candidate is invited to the interview.

Timeframe for interviews

A candidate selected for interview will be invited from November in their Year 13 until the end of January or later. This can vary depending on the medical school. There is no particular order for the invitation. From November, keep checking regularly both your UCAS account and the email address that you have registered with UCAS; please visit your spam or junk folder as some emails can land there. The candidate will be given a short timeframe to select the interview date and time slot, or may be offered an interview slot straightaway.

When to attend the interviews?

Each candidate has their own preferred style and attitude towards their preferred times for the interviews; however, the candidate may have less choice, as the medical school may give them a fixed slot. Most medical schools give a few options in a particular week; some give the option of three or four slots with a few weeks' gap; others just give one slot for the interview.

Remember that this is the busiest time when the candidate will be preparing for their final year A-level exams and some may have even started revision preparations. You may be lucky if the interviews come together in a particular week or within a short timeframe in either December or January of your Year 13. This way, you get to spend 2–3 weeks of intense preparation for interviews and then you will be able to focus on A-levels later. But if you get four interviews with lots of gaps in-between, prepare and then keep spending a small amount of time every week for interviews, while your focus is on your academic A-level subjects.

Selecting a time slot is important if you are given an option; if you are travelling from far away, it is wise for you to select a later morning or afternoon slot. The authors advise the candidate to arrive well ahead of time. Find a café or restaurant where you can go and relax and wind down calmly for at least half an hour before going for the interview. Traffic and parking conditions have to be taken into account and there is no point in getting stressed for these reasons just before the interview. If your interview is very early in the morning and if you are far away, it is worth finding a hotel or bed and breakfast accommodation near the venue and staying the previous night.

Attending the interview

Dress professionally and maintain good body language. Smile at the examiners but show empathy if you are role playing. Stay calm and structure the answer well. Selectors are looking for candidates who can show empathy, communicate well, and have a good attitude. It is important to display your motivation and awareness of the problems in healthcare.

Practise and revise well

Each medical school explicitly tells the candidate about the format and structure of the interviews when they are invited. MMIs usually have 6–8 stations on different themes. Prepare yourself and get lots of practice from friends/family, teachers/career guidance staff, and any advisers. Attending courses is helpful to get real-life practice; the authors recommend attending the national RISE charity MMI course run in the first or second week of November in Leicester. Further details are available from their website: www.risefoundationuk.com/mmi.

Practice, practice, and more practice

Interviews are easy to tackle if the candidate has had enough practice. Most interviews for the MMI will have 6–8 stations with a standard format including communication stations, role playing, stations on ethics, challenging scenarios, CV, work experience, etc. As these are the common ones, it is worth practising them repeatedly before going to the real interviews. One of the stations may be about recent health-related topics, but this can be answered if the candidate keeps track of BBC Health news and shows interest in listening to health-related news on other portals. There may be a mathematics/statistics/data analysis station, where a basic level of mathematics knowledge can help. Going to an interview practice course, and revising our MMI book mentioned at the beginning of this chapter will help; once you read the book, ask your parents, friends or well-wishers to ask the questions and see if you can answer the station or role play in 5–6 minutes.

Format of interviews

Most medical interviews are in the MMI formats, while a few still have panel interviews. The MMI format has 6–8 stations, each of 5–10 minutes, and runs for approximately 1 hour. Most of them have stations on communication, medical ethics, general ethics, personal qualities to demonstrate motivation, role play, NHS framework, and awareness of the structure/curriculum of their medical school/why they want to come to this medical school and the city. Some may have mathematics/data interpretation stations; some can have a station on their personal statement or work experience discussions. A few medical schools ask candidates to view a video and comment on the communication skills in the video. Some discuss recent health topics or chronic conditions and ask if the candidate has any opinion on how to manage them. The format varies and each medical school explains clearly about these on their websites.

Panel interviews are disappearing now, as they can be biased; these usually have two parts with two examiners each. The discussions in the panel are similar in topics to the MMI but there may not be any role-play stations. Usually they are approximately 30–60 minutes, although some differ.

In any of these interview formats, the interviewers are looking for a motivated candidate, who can communicate well, understands the career, and has good personal qualities. It is the duty of the candidate to demonstrate these during the interviews.

Structure of talking

Always introduce yourself with a smile. Good body language with eye contact, sitting straight, having hands in the right position, and reflecting on the question can help. Listen to what the examiner or actor says; read the question properly if you are given printed material or data, and think twice about what is asked.

When answering a station, there is a structured format that you need to follow:

1. Introduction (and checking if it is the right patient in role-play stations).
2. Opening statement (especially if an ethics station, summarise nicely with an opening statement).
3. Answer clearly without repetition. If it is an ethics station, talk clearly about the pros and cons of a particular situation.
4. Then express what your opinion is; you are not expected to solve an ethical dilemma, but the interviews expect that you are aware of the dilemma, and have your own opinion.
5. Closure — summarise the answer, or give your view of the dilemma. If it is a role-play station, conclude the station after asking 'Is there anything else you want to ask or want me to explain?'
6. Thank the examiner or the role-playing patient.

Three important tasks in interviews

There are three things that you should NOT forget:

1. You should quote the GMC's ethical guidance called *Good Medical Practice*. All ethical scenarios should be answered with awareness of this framework. If you quote this, you could achieve more marks for that section of the station.
2. Use the four pillars of medical ethics (autonomy, non-maleficence, beneficence and justice) to answer the question whenever possible; you may use one or more of these pillars to substantiate your answer on ethical scenarios.

3. Think about whether you can bring your work or volunteering experience into these answers. For example, if the question is about teamwork or communication skills in medicine, you should say how important it is, how it helps the outcome for the patient, and then quote an example from your previous work experience in which you observed this and realised its importance.

The authors have coached many candidates in the past and have realised that most candidates have prepared the first two points and have good work/volunteering experience, but forget to quote them in the actual interview. This could be due to the busy schedule of the MMI as well as the stress related to the interview; if the candidate has practised the answers many times, it will become more natural to address these three important points.

Ethical scenarios

Do not think that you need to solve the ethical dilemma; you just need to express your views from both sides, and then your own personal opinion. You should base your answers on the four pillars of medical ethics wherever possible:

1. Autonomy — giving respect to the patient and letting them make the decisions.
2. Non-maleficence — doing no harm.
3. Beneficence — always acting to benefit the patient.
4. Justice — consideration of the law and the overall benefit to society.

The GMC has published its ethical guidance called *Good Medical Practice* and the candidate is expected to know the four domains and the principles (available on their website: https://www.gmc-uk.org/ethical-guidance):

- Domain 1 — knowledge, skills and development:
  - providing a good standard of practice and care, and working within their competence;
  - keeping their knowledge and skills up to date.
- Domain 2 — patients, partnership and communication:
  - respecting every patient's dignity and treating them as individuals;

  - listening to patients and working in partnership with them, supporting them to make informed decisions about their care;
  - protecting the patient's personal information from improper disclosure.
- Domain 3 — colleagues, culture and safety:
  - working with colleagues in the best interests of the patients;
  - treating people with respect and creating a compassionate environment, where everyone feels safe to ask questions and raise concerns;
  - taking care of their own health and well-being.
- Domain 4 — trust and professionalism:
  - acting with honesty and integrity;
  - avoiding unfair discrimination against patients or colleagues.

Communication stations

Communication stations assess if the candidate can effectively convey information; listening skills are vital, and most MMIs assess this ability. Demonstrating empathy is very important in these stations. In role play, communication with challenging patients such as patients with dementia, or understanding the difficulties of family members of those with chronic medical problems, can be tested. It is vital that the candidate listens to the concerns, shows their empathy, reflects and allays their anxieties, assures them to get help or provides signposts for help. It is important that at the end the candidate concludes the station by asking: 'Is there anything else that you want to ask me?'

Curriculum of the medical school

Each medical school has a different curriculum and teaching style; some may have dissection while others may not. It is very important that the candidate has researched these well before attending the interview. The interviewer may test the candidate to see if they are really interested and have done their research before coming to the medical school. It is also important to know what other social and non-academic opportunities are available in that medical school and in the city where the candidate will be living for the next 5 years.

Patient safety

In all clinical scenarios, it is vital to stress that the candidate's goal will be to assure patient safety. Awareness of their own limitations and getting help from senior colleagues is vital.

Key Points

- **Most medical schools use an MMI format to assess prospective students.**
- **Communication and ethics stations should be prepared well as they are inevitable in these interviews.**
- **Use and quote the GMC's ethical guidance *Good Medical Practice*; be aware of the four domains of this guideline.**
- **Use the four pillars of medical ethics to support your answer on ethics; these include autonomy, non-maleficence, beneficence and justice.**
- **You should be explicit and volunteer the GMC guidance and four pillars of medical ethics whenever possible.**
- **Be sure to explain your work and volunteering experience when possible.**
- **Start practising early and attend the RISE MMI interview practice course at Leicester.**

References

1. General Medical Council. Good Medical Practice. The duties of medical professionals registered with the GMC. Available from: https://www.gmc-uk.org/professional-standards/the-professional-standards/good-medical-practice/the-duties-of-medical-professionals-registered-with-the-gmc.
2. Vasu T, Shyam S, RISE Foundation. *Interviews for Medical School: Multiple Mini Interview (MMI) Practice*. Shrewsbury, UK: tfm publishing; 2023.

Chapter 15

Results day for A-levels

Results day is one of the most important and stressful days for many A-level students. Usually the results will be released on a Thursday in the second or third week of August (earlier in Scotland). Students can collect their results from their college or school from 08:00 hours British Summer Time onwards; this could change to online results delivery very soon as per the future plans by the Government. Some schools and exam boards already deliver results by email or online for A-level examinations.

Some students may travel far during the college or school holidays after their Year 13 but the authors advise them to come back before the results day as it can be an experience for you to enjoy if you have the expected results; if you do not get the expected results, you need to do a few things on the day to look at alternative options, which are detailed later in this chapter and in the following two chapters.

Conditional offers

Medical schools offer conditional placements after the interviews; this means that the candidate has to achieve particular grades in their A-levels in three subjects. If you have taken four subjects, you can take the best three provided they are accepted by the medical school (see Chapter 6 for details of subjects). Most of the universities require A*AA while some require AAA and a very few require A*A*A. It is ideal for the candidate to aim for at least A*AA. Some candidates will not achieve the required or predicted grades despite passing through the UCAT exams with good scores and doing well in the interviews. Unfortunately, they will not be offered the places in the medical schools and will have to look at alternate plans (see Chapter 17) or look at the clearing system (see Chapter 16).

UCAS platform

The UCAS web platform updates the results and university offers at approximately 08:15 hours on the same day (there may be a delay due to the huge number of candidates). Universities receive the A-level results earlier and start sending email confirmation offers from 08:00 hours on the same day.

Collecting results from the school/college

This can be a stressful time, as your future career will be evident at that moment; if you prefer, take one of your parents with you. Parents can also be stressed. While standing in the queue, there may be moments of joy from previous students in the queue when they receive their results envelope, which may make you more anxious. Sleep well the previous night and try to do some breathing exercises before you go to the school or college. We suggest going in at 08:00 hours or slightly before, as there will be a queue of students waiting for the results; schools have experience of this and they may arrange tables in alphabetical order of names to make this process quick.

We advise going early as, if there is any problem, you could look at clearing options (see Chapter 16), although it is difficult to get medicine courses; this is to look at other allied courses rather than medicine. If you have not received any offers after the interviews, and if you achieve good grades, the clearing system will help you to locate another quick interview and place; candidates have done this and succeeded. If you had one place which needed A*A*A and you did not achieve these grades but received AAA, still the clearing system can help you to secure a place in a different medical school that accepts these grades (see Chapter 16 for further details).

What if you did not get through the interviews?

Some candidates may not have done well in the interviews and not received any offers; some may have applied to the wrong medical schools, which had different criteria from yours for the selection process. In these situations, the clearing system can help, but this may have opened up medical school places even a few weeks before the A-level results date and could have offered interviews. Provided your predicted grades are good, you should look out for these places in the UCAS web portal even a few days before the A-level results if you have had no interviews up to that point. If you apply, the medical schools will offer a quick interview or telephone interview and may offer you a place if successful; but this will still be conditional based on the required A-level grades.

The time near A-level results day is crucial if you have received no offers. If possible, it is wise to search the clearing system and think of a few options ready before the results day. Once you are prepared, we hope that you may not need to use the clearing system and you achieve the grades needed successfully.

Contacts after the results day

The UCAS phone lines will be busy on results day although they appoint many extra advisers on that day. You should prepare and seek out their contact details ready before the results day.

You could also write down the contact details of the medical schools and the fifth choice that you made, if you need to contact them after the results. We hope that you achieve what you expected with the grades but, every year, there are a few candidates who do not succeed; this chapter and the following two chapters are to help them, as it can be a difficult day for them.

Nominating a person

If you are not there to collect the results on the results day or if you do not want to collect them, you can nominate a person to collect them at the school or college, or you can check if the results can be received online.

With the UCAS, you can also nominate another person to speak on your behalf on the results day.

Unexpected grades

If you receive unexpected grades it is unfortunate but, apart from clearing systems and the other options, you should speak to the teacher or adviser at the school or college. They can advise and guide you with the next steps.

You can speak to the college or university and see if they can be flexible. The options are very limited for a career in medicine, but there may be some instances when they can be of help. For example, if you have done an EPQ and have good scores, they may consider it. There is no guarantee but it is worth liaising immediately with the admissions team in the medical school.

You may wish to appeal your grades to the exam boards. The authors know of candidates who have been successful in getting a higher grade with an appeal after they had been borderline with a lower grade. However, talk to the medical school admissions team immediately and let them know that you are applying for an appeal against the received grades. They may not wait, but at least you have made them aware. The authors have heard of scenarios in which the candidate received higher grades, but it was late as the places were filled for that year; however, the medical school accepted the candidate to take the course for the following year (which means a gap year before the course starts).

If the candidate wants to appeal against their grades, they should first talk to the college or school; they will look at the options and then submit a request to the exam board on behalf of the candidate. The candidates can themselves also appeal directly to the awarding organisation, which will send you a final report after they have reviewed the result. The exam board will check your answer papers for marking mistakes; your marks may change if there are any. Please remember that the new grade could be the same or higher or even lower than the original after the appeal.

Preparing for the results day

The authors advise preparing for the A-level results day beforehand:

- Keep your UCAS ID and login details safe. Check they are working a day or two before the results.
- Keep a record of the hotline numbers or contact details of all the medical school admissions teams that you have applied for, or have had offers from. Keep the contact details of the UCAS team and the clearing team.
- Charge your mobile phone fully before you go for the results; have the phone charger available if you need to call the universities. There will be a long wait and be prepared for it.
- Have a notepad and pen ready to jot down numbers and details.
- It may be wise to save a copy of your personal statement and GCSE results in an easily reachable folder on your computer.
- Once you have prepared all these steps, we hope that you will not need to use them on your results day.

Key Points

- **The A-level results day can be stressful and the candidate should prepare well for this day.**
- **We advise the candidate to take a parent with them.**
- **Please remember your UCAS login details.**
- **It is wise to keep contact details of the UCAS and the applied medical schools admission teams, if you need them.**
- **If you achieve unexpected grades, do not panic; there may be other options available.**

References

1. UCAS. Unexpected grades. Available from: https://www.ucas.com/applying/after-you-apply/clearing-and-results-day/results-day/unexpected-grades.
2. UK Government. Gov.uk. Appeal against a GCSE, AS or A-level grade or the result of a qualification. Available from: https://www.gov.uk/appeal-qualification-result.
3. Universities and Colleges Admissions Service (UCAS). Results day. Available from: https://www.ucas.com/applying/after-you-apply/clearing-and-results-day/results-day.

Chapter 16

Clearing system in the UCAS

UCAS uses a clearing system that helps to fill the places that are still available in the medical schools after allocations. This could be due to various reasons: some students may have had more than two offers and they have to decline the excess offers in June; some students who have two offers would take one as firm and keep one as insurance, and when they drop the second choice, they may go for clearing; some students change their mind and decline the offer of medical schools. Universities estimate these numbers based on their past experience but they may get some unfilled places and these are opened to the clearing system. The clearing usually happens after the main application cycle has concluded.

The clearing system also helps students who did not achieve the needed grades in their A-level examinations; they may opt to choose other subjects with their lower grades.

When can you use clearing?

In general, clearing opens from 5th July and continues until 20th October in that year. You can use clearing if:

- You did not receive any offers; usually this means that you can apply for subjects other than medicine. Some students will be offered medicine at a different medical school provided their required minimum grades are achieved.

- You want to apply for non-medical courses if you are applying late in the UCAS system.
- You did not meet the conditions of your offers.
- You have declined your firm place in the UCAS hub.

Clearing after results days

If you did not get the expected grades on the results day, you can add a clearing choice in the UCAS hub from 13:00 hours on the A-level results day.

Ask for advice

It is worth talking to your adviser at school or college, or liaising with the careers office. You can also talk to the UCAS hotline, as well as individual admissions teams from different medical schools, to see if there are places depending on your grades. When you contact individual universities, it is better to enquire about their specific requirements.

When you contact UCAS or universities, please have your UCAS ID number, clearing number (if available), and your academic details to answer the questions of the admissions team. It is wise to take a notepad and jot down the names and phone numbers of different medical schools or other subject courses in universities, and also have the course code and title. The phone lines may be busy on results day, so sit in a quiet area where the mobile phone signal is good.

Medical school places are limited

Most medical schools do not enter clearing; only a few enter as the spaces are limited for medicine and are highly competitive.

Be prepared to act swiftly

There are only limited medical school places for clearing; if you have an option, be prepared to act quickly. You may need to attend a telephone interview or an online interview immediately. You may have to make decisions swiftly. It is wise to do some research on the medical schools to which you might apply for clearing if there is an opportunity.

Things to keep ready

You will need a few things to prepare for the clearing system:

- Pen and a notepad to jot down details and contact numbers.
- Quiet area with good telephone and Wi-Fi signal.
- UCAS ID, personal details.
- GCSE and A-level results.
- Personal statement.
- A fully charged phone and laptop, and have the charger ready.
- Good professional clothes, if you are called for an interview on the same day (and have someone to drive you if possible).

Calling the university on results day

Some medical schools offer places to those who were not offered interviews, but this comes out of clearing. It is worth contacting the universities to which you had applied to see if they have any spaces available.

Courses other than medicine

Clearing helps candidates to secure a place in related or other courses if they have not been offered a place in medical school. Many candidates choose Biomedical Sciences, Biotechnology or Biological Sciences courses; this could be an entirely different degree thus moving forward in an alternative direction. Another option would be to do this degree first and then apply to medicine via graduate entry (see Chapter 20).

Courses other than medicine could be easily available from clearing as they may have lower cut-off requirements for grades compared with medicine, but this does not apply to all courses and also depends on the particular university. It is worth looking at the website of the universities for other courses, their minimum requirements, and then phoning or contacting them immediately.

It is important to research the universities and courses that could interest you before the results day and make a list of potential options. Clearing operates on a first-come, first-served basis, although there may be phone, online, or in-person interviews.

Facts about clearing from medical schools

There is no guarantee for clearing spaces, but the authors have noted that few medical schools offer clearing every year. You have to be flexible and look for all options.

The medical schools do not lower their academic standards or minimum required grades during clearing; they only give another option for an interview and the other practicalities. Even with the UCAT, they expect a good score. The candidate should also attend an interview.

The candidate should not reject any available offers from a medical school with the hope of clearing in the future from a different medical school, as there is no guarantee that clearing will happen. Even if a medical school has offered clearing in the previous year, this might not be offered in the next year. Getting a place in medical school is very competitive and the authors recommend proper research and a systematic approach for applications.

Key Points

- **The clearing system helps to fill places that are not filled in the medical schools; as medicine is highly competitive, there are only a few chances to succeed in this.**
- **Still, it is worth trying if you have all the minimum requirements for that particular medical school.**
- **Proper research and being prepared will help before using the clearing system.**
- **If you are happy to take a course other than medicine, the clearing system can help you with many options.**

References

1. UCAS. Clearing and results day. Available from: https://www.ucas.com/applying/after-you-apply/clearing-and-results-day.

Chapter 17

What if you are not lucky this time?

Unfortunately, medical school placement is extremely competitive with approximately 15–20 applications being received for each place. Proper research, planning, hard work and a systematic approach can help you to secure a place in medical school. However, if you do not get offered a place, it is not the end of the world. There are various options still available and this chapter details them. The authors really hope that the readers will not need these pathways and are successful in their first attempt.

Do not panic or get frustrated

Every year, there are many students who do not succeed in their application to medical school. This can be devastating for both students and their parents, especially if they had been given a conditional offer from the medical school of their choice and this failed due to unexpected grades at A-levels. Please do not panic or get frustrated as this happens to some students every year and you are not alone. It is important to be calm and composed, and think of the next plans and work towards them.

Options available

If you did not succeed in getting a place in medical school this time, the options are:

- Look at the clearing options and see if there is any possibility (Chapter 16).
- Take another related course and apply through the graduate entry course for medicine (Chapter 20).
- Apply to study medicine abroad; most of the students in this pathway go to Europe (Chapter 19).
- Pathway degrees for a guaranteed medicine interview.
- Apply for the apprenticeship pathway for medicine (Chapter 18).
- Move towards allied health-related courses.
- Resit A-level exams and try medicine next year.
- Take a gap year and think over your plans again.

Research and analyse

Having a plan B can help if a candidate is not successful, but many students do not do this. It is essential to research and talk to many people, including your parents, friends, teachers, career advisers, and other advisers. In the end, if you are not successful, you do not want to get stuck on a course or career that you do not enjoy.

Studying abroad in medical school

Every year, hundreds of students move towards Europe to study medicine. The conditions of living, course curriculum, fee structure, and language challenges can all vary depending on the country and university; the student has to do their research and look at all the options. See Chapter 19 for further details.

Graduate entry for medical school

This may look like a straightforward pathway, but there are challenges including the difficulties in getting a place after graduation. Furthermore, it can take a long time, and the entry criteria are different. Only a few medical schools have this option. The financial burden of another 3–4 years of university life has also to be considered. See Chapter 20 for details.

Pathway degrees

Some universities such as Swansea offer pathway degrees; these offer students the opportunity of a guaranteed interview for graduate entry medicine. Some candidates may prefer to choose this as their fifth choice in the UCAS application. However, there is no guarantee that you will succeed in the interview unless you work hard to fulfil the minimum requirements for the graduate entry medicine pathway (see Chapter 20).

Apprenticeship course for medicine

The UK Government has recently introduced the apprenticeship pathway to become a doctor. The programme outcome has yet to be seen but this could be an option for those who want to be in the UK and do not want to waste a year. See Chapter 18 for details.

Allied healthcare profession

Some medical schools offer places in other allied health science subjects to those who were not successful in getting into medicine, but this can also come out of the clearing system. It is worth calling universities to which you applied to see if they have any spaces available.

These could include but are not limited to: pharmacy, physiotherapy, nursing, occupational therapy, optometry, radiography, speech and language therapy, operating department practice, paramedic work, dietetics, and other allied roles. Some also move towards healthcare management, medical journalism, public health, genetics, research, etc.

Resit for A-level exams

If you do not get the needed grades for going to a medical school, you could resit the A-level exams at a later date. Some universities do not accept resits and it is wise to check which universities accept them before applying in the following year. Some may also have limitations on the number of resits.

Some universities offer foundation courses or gateway courses, with one extra year to strengthen academic knowledge; this may also be needed if you have not taken the science subject that the university recommends. However, the spaces are very limited and difficult to obtain.

Students can resit A-level exams in their own school or college or as external candidates at exam centres. You should resit exams only if you can improve your grades with an extra year of learning; however, it is wise to get some work experience part-time to improve your personal statement and interview skills at the same time.

The risks of retaking exams are: you may get a lower grade or the same grade, you will spend one more year studying, you will be one year behind your peers, and you will have to pay fees to resit exams. You cannot resit exams in November like some GCSEs but you have to do it the following year in May/June.

Gap year before medical school

You may wish to take a gap year before medical school if you were not successful; you could use this time to gain work experience and interview practice; or you could use this time to gain better UCAT exam scores. If your UCAT scores have been low, and your grades are very good, it may be worth getting some work experience and retaking the UCAT exam, but remember that you will have to go through the interviews again.

Key Points

- Medical school places are very competitive; you are not alone if you do not succeed this time.
- There are a variety of options if you are not successful.
- You could think of applying to a medical school abroad in Europe.
- The step forward depends on your personal situation; we strongly advise you to discuss options with your teachers, family and career advisers as soon as possible.

References

1. UCAS. Medicine. Available from: https://www.ucas.com/explore/subjects/medicine.
2. Swansea University. Pathways to medicine. Available from: https://www.swansea.ac.uk/medicine/pathways/.

Chapter 18

Medical doctor degree apprenticeships

NHS England introduced a new medical doctor degree apprenticeship from September 2024, as part of the Long Term Workforce Plan. It is too early to assess the efficacy and outcome of this programme, but it could be a pathway for those who have not succeeded in getting a medical school place. The future of this pilot scheme is not yet clear, but it has been added to this book for the sake of completeness.

Apprenticeships

There are advantages in this pathway: apprentices will earn a wage while training and they do not need to pay any tuition fees. The pilot scheme started in September 2024. The Government has assured the profession that these apprenticeship trainees will need to meet the same high standards as those who do a traditional medical school undergraduate degree. They will meet all the criteria set out by the GMC. They will attend a medical school to complete an accredited medical degree.

Recruitment

The UK Government has introduced this scheme to recruit more frontline medics to the NHS. However, doubts exist as to whether this will set lower standards and a different pathway with a two-tiered doctor system. The

Government hopes that it will bring people from different backgrounds into the medical profession, and who will be more representative of the local communities.

Curriculum

It is too early to comment on the curriculum, but the Government has assured that these apprenticeship candidates will have the same academic qualifications as those who complete their degree through medical school. The apprenticeship will typically last 5 years and the candidates have to complete the Medical Licensing Assessment (MLA) examination.

Applying for the apprenticeships

These medical doctor apprenticeships will be advertised through NHS Jobs (https://www.jobs.nhs.uk/candidate) periodically or via the Government's Find an apprenticeship website (https://www.gov.uk/apply-apprenticeship).

Future of the apprenticeships

The future of the apprenticeship schemes is not clear at this stage as the Government announced this as a pilot project. The authors are not sure if this will continue in the future; the NHS England website mentions that the funding was available only for cohorts from 2024 and 2025.

Key Points

- **In September 2024, the UK Government started an apprenticeship medical degree programme as a pilot project.**
- **We are not sure if this will continue in the future.**

References

1. Gov.UK. Blog. The Education Hub. Medical doctor apprenticeships: everything you need to know; 5th February 2024. Available from: https://educationhub.blog.gov.uk/2024/02/nhs-doctor-apprenticeships-everything-you-need-to-know/.
2. NHS England. Workforce, training and education. Medical doctor degree apprenticeship. Available from: https://www.hee.nhs.uk/our-work/talent-care-widening-participation/apprenticeships/medical-doctor-degree-apprenticeship.

Chapter 19

Applications to universities abroad

Studying medicine abroad should not be seen as a last resort. Many countries across Europe offer high-quality teaching at reasonable prices and are a great option. Not only can you pursue a medical career, but it also comes with the benefit of being able to experience a different culture.

However, it is important to acknowledge the fierce competition and that thousands of students are unsuccessful in their applications to medical schools in the UK. There are multiple different options for students in this situation, including studying a different course, taking a gap year or pursuing a medical degree in another country.

The challenges of studying abroad

Although grade requirements may be lower than those required for the UK medical schools, it is still challenging to get a medical seat abroad. Most universities have separate entrance exams for core sciences and English Language skills. Although the course itself may be taught in English, medical students are expected to be able to interact fully with patients, so you should be ready to learn the local language.

Acclimatising to the new atmosphere while keeping up with the intense coursework can be tough. There are many differences between studying medicine in the UK and abroad in Europe. For example, the teaching is likely to be more traditional and the course is usually 6 years long rather than 5.

Most UK student loans do not cover foreign education, so financing the degree may be a challenge as well. Conversely, tuition fees may be reasonable and many European options may have a lower cost of living than the UK.

Some universities may ask for transcripts of your certificates (legalised and translated) in their local language; there will be directions on their website on how to get these as per the requirements.

UKMLA examination

In the past, candidates who had trained in Europe or abroad had to take the Professional and Linguistic Assessments Board (PLAB) test to get a licence from the GMC to practice in the UK. Now, even students studying in the UK have to take the MLA examination before getting a GMC licence to practice; the same rule also applies to those trained in Europe. However, students from medical schools in the UK may be well prepared for this UKMLA examination as the curriculum focuses on this examination.

Facts to check from medical schools abroad

When choosing the correct course for you, there are many things to look for:

- Is the course recognised by the GMC? To practice in the UK, the GMC must accept the medical degree. Make sure to check the GMC's website and see if the university is accepted.
- Is the entire course taught in English? Studying medicine in a new language is nearly impossible. It may also be helpful if the university provides local language training in preparation for communicating with patients in later years.
- What are the entry requirements? Usually universities require students to have qualifications in the core sciences. They may also require an entrance exam, which will require separate preparation.

- Are the entrance exams online? Most universities have arrangements for students to take entrance exams online, but some require you to travel to a test centre.
- Are the costs manageable? Make sure to check the annual tuition fees and the cost of living. There may also be some hidden fees involved with the application process.
- Does the university have a good reputation?
- Are there any post-graduation pathways? You need to research the options after graduation. Is it possible to return to the UK or enter residency elsewhere?
- Student feedback. A quick Google search can reveal important reviews from previous students who were in the same situation as you. Teaching quality, facilities and living conditions are very important.

We have compiled a list of some popular medical schools in Europe which offer education in English. It is important to note that this information is subject to change every academic year. It should be used as a framework to decide what options are available but please make sure to do your own research in addition.

Medical schools in Poland

Medical University of Warsaw

- Website: https://www.wum.edu.pl/studies-in-english.
- One of the top-ranked medical universities in Poland.
- Offers a 6-year course in English.
- Entrance exams in Biology, Chemistry and Physics are required unless the student has sat the BMAT, MCAT, GAMSAT or UCAT exam.
- Foundation year course available.
- Tuition fees: €17,100 per year for 6 years.

Jagiellonian University Medical College (Krakow)

- Website: https://medschool.uj.edu.pl/.
- Six-year programme in English.
- Biology or Physics and Chemistry courses completed during secondary education (A-levels).

- Admissions are based solely on entrance exam results (held online for 2025/2026 applicants).
- Tuition fees: €15,500 per year for 6 years.

Medical schools in Cyprus

University of Nicosia Medical School

- Website: https://www.unic.ac.cy/med.
- Six-year course taught in English.
- ABB in A-levels, Biology and one more science subject needed.
- An online interview is used for assessment.
- Tuition fees: €22,000 per year.

European University Cyprus School of Medicine

- Website: https://euc.ac.cy/en/academics/schools-departments/school-of-medicine/.
- Six-year course in English.
- Tuition fees: €23,000 per year.

Medical schools in Hungary

Semmelweis University Medical School, Budapest

- Website: https://semmelweis.hu/admission/programs/medicine/.
- Six-year course in English.
- Entrance exam in Biology, Chemistry, English and Biomedical English.
- The interview also includes an oral examination to assess the applicant's knowledge.
- Tuition fees: US$9950 per semester, for a total of 12 semesters.

University of Debrecen Medical School

- Website: https://aok.unideb.hu/.
- Six-year course in English.
- The entrance exam also tests English Language proficiency.
- Tuition fees: US$16,950 per year.

Medical schools in Malta

Queen Mary University of London (in Malta)

- Website: https://www.qmul.ac.uk/malta/.
- A similar programme to the MBBS programme in London.
- Five-year course in English.
- A-level grades of AAA in Biology, Chemistry, Mathematics or Physics (in one sitting).
- GCSE grades of AAABBB (7, 7, 7, 6, 6, 6) in Biology, Chemistry, English Language, and Mathematics in any order.
- UCAT score of 2281 or above in the last year.
- Prospective students will need to participate in the interview phase.
- Tuition fees: €37,500 per year.

Medical schools in Czechia

First Faculty of Medicine Charles University, Prague

- Website: https://en.lf1.cuni.cz/applicants.
- A-levels are not required but you must pass entrance exams in Biology, Chemistry and Physics.
- Six-year course in English.
- The university has multiple faculties of medicine. Each has its own teaching style and focus.
- Entrance exam tests Biology, Chemistry and Physics. There is also an MMI format.
- Tuition fees: €24,250 per year.

Faculty of Medicine Masaryk University

- Website: https://www.muni.cz/en/bachelors-and-masters-study-programmes/study-at-faculty-of-medicine.
- Separate entrance exams on Chemistry, Biology and Physics. E-learning preparatory course available.
- Taught in English but an intensive Czech language preparatory course is offered.
- Six-year course in English.
- Tuition fees: Kč 380,000 CZK (approx €15,500 per year — rates can vary).

- A-level grades of AAB in Chemistry, Biology, Physics or Mathematics, respectively.

Medical schools in Bulgaria

Medical University of Sofia

- Website: https://mu-sofia.bg/en/admission/admissions-of-foreign-citizen/.
- Six-year course in English.
- Documents/certificates need to be translated into Bulgarian by approved translators.
- Admissions test for Biology, Chemistry and English Language.
- Tuition fees: €9950 per year.

Medical University of Plovdiv

- Website: https://mu-plovdiv.bg/en/admission-info/admission-to-english-taught-programmes/specialties-and-application-deadline/.
- Translation and legalisation of documents/certificates needed.
- Online entrance exam for Biology, Chemistry and English Language; examples of test papers available on their website.
- Six-year course taught in English.
- Tuition fees: €9000 per year and €8000 for the final year.

Medical schools in Romania

Carol Davila University of Medicine and Pharmacy (Bucharest)

- Website: https://umfcd.ro/studenti/viitori-studenti/.
- Six-year course taught in English.
- 75% pass required in Biology and Chemistry at A-level.
- Online interview stage (assesses science topics too).
- Tuition fees: €10,000 per year.

Grigore T. Popa University of Medicine and Pharmacy (Iași)

- Website: https://www.umfiasi.ro/ro.
- Six-year course in English, with only three foreign places.
- Not sure if GMC approved.

- No entrance exam.
- Academic record is important.
- Tuition fees: €8400 per year.

Iuliu Hațieganu University of Medicine and Pharmacy (Cluj-Napoca)

- Website: https://umfcluj.ro/en/.
- Six-year course taught in English.
- No entrance exam.
- Admission score calculated from academic performance in A-levels.
- Tuition fees: €10,000 for the first year, reducing gradually to €6000 in the sixth year.

Medical schools in Greece

University of Crete School of Medicine

- Website: https://imed.med.uoc.gr/admissions/.
- Six-year course in English.
- A-levels in Chemistry, Biology and one more science subject needed.
- MCAT and UCAT are accepted for assessment.
- Interviews will be online.
- Tuition fees: €15,000 per year.

Medical schools in Georgia

- There are many medical schools in Georgia where UK students are studying.
- The curriculum and pattern vary.
- Fees are between €3800 and €7000 per year.

This is not a full list of medical schools available in Europe, but only a snapshot. We suggest you look at their websites as the details can change periodically. Furthermore, there are many universities on other continents that some may be interested in. We could not add all of them here as there are too many to list. It is recommended that a candidate does extensive research online if they are considering studying abroad.

We advise liaising with the career advisers, university representatives, and speaking to previous and present students to get an idea about the medical school, living conditions, curriculum and the clinical facilities before you decide on this pathway. It may be worth travelling to the university to check whether the culture and values of the city and medical school will suit you.

Important disclaimer

We strongly urge candidates to carry out their own due diligence and proper research before applying to these universities. It is advisable for candidates and their parents to visit the city and the university before making a decision as they will be spending their next 6 years there.

Key Points

- **Do the research if you are planning to go abroad to study in a medical school.**
- **Check if the medical school is GMC recognised.**
- **Be prepared to learn about the local language and culture.**
- **Entrance requirements and assessments vary between different countries.**
- **Be prepared to take the UKMLA exam once you finish your medical school if you wish to practise in the UK.**

References

1. General Medical Council: Medical Licensing Assessment. Available from: https://www.gmc-uk.org/education/medical-licensing-assessment.

Chapter 20

Graduate entry for medicine

Graduate entry medicine (GEM) programmes are offered by some medical schools only; this is a faster route to get a medical degree if you are already a graduate with a degree. This is a 4-year programme compared with the traditional 5-year medical school programme after A-levels. Participants receive the same degree and have the same pathway to register with the GMC to get a practice licence.

Competition for GEM

Only a few medical schools offer this and it can be highly competitive. Universities such as Warwick, Swansea, Nottingham, Surrey, St George's, King's College, etc. offer a GEM pathway. At present, Warwick (203 places), Swansea (150 places), Nottingham and St George's have more medical school places for the GEM pathway while others only have a few places.

UCAS application

The GEM application process is similar to any other undergraduate course via UCAS (see Chapter 11). The UCAS code for GEM is A101. You are only allowed to apply to four medical schools and do not have a fifth choice as for the traditional entry, as you have already completed a graduate degree.

Entry criteria

Entry criteria vary between different medical schools and it is best to check their website. Some universities even accept non-science graduate degrees for this pathway.

Academic performance

The minimum requirement for most GEM courses is a 2:1 degree, which is an upper second class honours degree. This is a high academic performance with a 60–70% average score.

Aptitude tests

You need to check the medical school website for the requirements; some universities ask for the Graduate Medical School Admissions Test (GAMSAT) exam, while others use the same UCAT exam, as for the traditional route.

Interviews

As in the traditional pathway, GEM entry also requires good performance in the interviews, which have similar expectations and standards.

Work experience

Being a graduate and mature candidate, some medical schools expect work experience and this can be checked from their website.

Research thoroughly

As the options are limited and the places are very competitive, a candidate interested in the GEM pathway should carry out extensive research and be focused on the application process. It is prudent to check the university and medical school websites to plan early and keep checking for their application and entry criteria.

GEM in Europe

Graduate entry courses are also available in many European countries; they use GAMSAT, Medical College Admission Test (MCAT) or UCAT along with interviews to select the candidates.

Pathway degrees

Some universities such as Swansea offer pathway degrees; these offer students the opportunity of a guaranteed interview for GEM. For this reason, some candidates may prefer to choose this as their fifth choice in the UCAS application, while applying during their A-levels. However, there is no guarantee that you will succeed in the interview unless you work hard to fulfil minimum requirements for the GEM pathway.

The medical school will expect a few standards for this pathway; for example, Swansea University expects these candidates to achieve a 60% average in Year 1 to be eligible to take the pathways module in Year 2. They have to achieve 60% in a specific module in Year 2. They should get good scores in the aptitude tests. They can only use the interview guarantee once, in their final year of study.

Is GEM the right option?

The authors feel that the GEM option is only suited for those who are highly motivated to go towards medicine and are prepared to work hard in their degree course to get a 2:1 score; they also have to achieve good scores in aptitude tests and do well in the interviews. There are hundreds of candidates who succeed in this pathway every year.

Key Points

- **The GEM programme is a 4-year course for degree holders to become doctors.**
- **You have to achieve good grades in your degree course, score well in aptitude tests, and do well in interviews.**
- **Check with the medical school website for the minimum requirements and the entry criteria.**

References

1. Swansea University. Medicine (Graduate Entry), MBBCH. Available from: https://www.swansea.ac.uk/undergraduate/courses/medicine/medicine-graduate-entry-mbbch/#entry-requirements=is-expanded.
2. Swansea University. Pathways to Medicine. Available from: https://www.swansea.ac.uk/medicine/pathways/.
3. University of Warwick. Warwick Medical School. Graduate Entry Medicine (MBChB). Available from: https://warwick.ac.uk/fac/sci/med/study/ugr/.

Chapter 21

Taking care of physical health

Preparing for entry to a medical school in Years 12 and 13 can be tiring and daunting for many. It can make you feel overwhelmed, stressed and add pressure to your academic performance if it is not balanced properly. At the same time, many parents can become stressed with the sheer amount of overwhelming information about medical school entry. It is vital that you take care of your physical and mental health whilst studying for your A-levels.

A healthy mind and healthy body are both vital; for the sake of ease, we have split this into two chapters — Chapters 21 and 22. The authors strongly recommend that you read both chapters together.

Physical health

Without a healthy body, you cannot perform well in your A-level or medical school assessments. Suitable nutrition with a healthy balanced diet, good sleep, regular exercise and a balanced lifestyle are vital for success.

Nutrition and hydration

Healthy eating, a balanced diet, and sufficient hydration are essential. Candidates can easily forget to drink enough water and suffer from dehydration and headaches during the busy school or college time or during revision. Make sure that you drink at least 1.5–2 litres of water every day; this can vary depending on the climate, activities and your overall health. We suggest using a marked water bottle as you can easily forget during the busy schedule in A-levels. A balanced diet is essential with enough protein to take care of your teenage growth needs. Plenty of fruits and vegetables (at least five portions per day) are advised for a healthy body, which helps you to concentrate on your studies. Adolescent girls may not get enough iron and are advised to eat red meat, liver, spinach and whole grains.

Eat an adequate number of whole grains, lean protein and dairy products, while avoiding sugary and processed foods, and unhealthy fats. Eating balanced meals at regular times and healthy snacks to maintain energy during a busy day is advised. Do not skip meals, especially breakfast. Limit caffeine and sugary drinks as this can increase anxiety levels significantly.

Good sleep

It is busy for you during A-levels and medical school preparations, and you may feel that no amount of time is enough; but getting 8 hours of sleep per night allows you to recover and concentrate on studies the next day. Establishing a regular sleeping time improves your sleep pattern. Sleep helps to improve memory and cognition. There is good scientific evidence to show that good sleep hygiene also improves your immunity and hormonal control.

Having a calming schedule before bed can help, such as a warm bath, reading, listening to gentle music, etc. Try avoiding your phone or electronic devices just before going to bed as the blue light can interfere with the regulation of sleep.

Regular exercise

Routine exercise and physical activity help to boost your mood and help you to focus on your studies. Your mood levels also improve with exercise. Aim for at least 30 minutes of walking or moderate exercise for at least 5 days a week.

Sports

If you play a sport or take part in martial arts or gymnastics, try to go for at least one session every week. Your local sports club in that particular sport may have a weekly squad for teenagers. It will give you a moral boost, as well as a way to let go of your stress. It may also help with your social life and mood.

Joining a local gym can help; going at least 2 or 3 days a week can help you unwind your stress. It will also help to build up your muscle strength. Swimming helps to refresh you if there are facilities available.

Short breaks between busy work periods

Sitting continuously in front of a computer while revising and studying can tire you and also affect your core muscle strength. In such situations, take regular breaks and your productivity will increase. Even a simple walk to a nearby shop, doing some stretching exercises in your garden, or a quick jog may help you to refresh and return to your study.

Get help early

If your health is affected, please speak to your GP and get help early. Without good health, you will not be able to focus on your A-level subjects.

Key Points

- **A healthy body will help you to focus and prepare for your A-level examinations.**
- **Adequately balanced nutrition and hydration are vital.**
- **Good sleep hygiene is vital to improving your memory and concentration.**
- **Get help early if your health is affected.**

References

1. NHS. Physical activity guidelines for children and young people. Available from: https://www.nhs.uk/live-well/exercise/physical-activity-guidelines-children-and-young-people/.

Chapter 22

Taking care of mental health

Preparing for medical school can be really stressful. Multiple examinations, interviews, aptitude tests, and application processes — all these can be compounded significantly, and affect your mood. The expectations from teachers/school/college as well as from parents can add to this stress. The stress levels of young adolescents are very high during the GCSE and A-level years.

This chapter should be read with the previous chapter on physical health (Chapter 21) as we have covered many vital topics such as regular exercise, sleep hygiene, nutrition and sufficient hydration, which are also important for mental health. We have not repeated them here to avoid duplication.

Managing a routine

Starting preparation early and having a regular routine will help to avoid stressful situations at the last minute. Having a timetable that is regularly reviewed and updated is important. Sometimes, you may lag behind in your timetable; accept that this is normal, and review and re-plan again. Small steps back do not mean failure and this is an opportunity to think ahead.

Time management

An A-level is a 2-year course, and most of the important academic topics are covered in Year 12 itself. Please make revision notes as you have to face exams only at the end of Year 13; appropriate preparation avoids stress and low mood. Accepting fall-backs in your plans and committing to future rescheduled plans are the way forward.

Rather than working on large tasks, try to split them into smaller chunks; this will keep you to your time schedule. Sometimes, you may want to plan your revision timetable in such a way that you rotate between different subjects to avoid boredom in a single topic or subject. Build regular breaks in your schedule to avoid burnout, and try to take regular breaks for exercise.

Setting realistic goals is important; you can become stressed if the goals are not achievable. Think well before making a timetable or plan; if it is not going as per the schedule, accept it and try to revise the plan with realistic goals.

Study strategies

Each student has their own best study technique; some like reading continuously, some like to make links with online resources, some like to write down points as they read. Techniques vary a lot, but it is important that you research what suits you and practise that technique.

Revision strategies

Revision is the key; most students become stressed during this time as they feel that there are too many topics to cover. First, feel confident that you have attended this topic in class; then, recollect what you have read after the class. It is prudent to make revision notes right from the beginning of Year 12. All high street stationery shops and online shops sell revision cards; writing down important points on these cards and looking at them later may help with revision and avoid stress nearer the exam time.

The most important step for success in preparation for A-level exams is to practise as many past exam papers as possible. Your teacher or school or college can help you to obtain these past papers. Your exam board website will have all past papers, which can be easily accessed. Make sure that you practise in real exam simulated timings and settings to prepare you to avoid stress during the exams.

Be positive

It is easily possible that you can lose confidence nearer the time of exams or interviews. Tell yourself that you have worked hard and focus on your strengths. A positive attitude and approach are the most important qualities for success in preparing for medical school.

Avoid negative beliefs

Many candidates preparing for medical school can keep worrying about the consequences of failing to get a place in medicine. They may feel that their life is a failure; this is not true. It is important that you work hard to get into a medical school, but it is not the end of the world if you did not get in that year. Anxiety about exams, interviews and application processes can make you stressed, which can significantly impair your performance. You should focus on what you can do rather than what you cannot do.

Replace these negative beliefs with positive beliefs. For example, if your negative belief is 'I am not good at organic chemistry', you could replace it with: 'even though organic chemistry is difficult for me, I am good at other subjects in chemistry; I do have a revision plan for organic chemistry and will stick to it and do better'.

Avoid comparison

Do not judge yourself against your friends or colleagues; everyone works in different ways and at different paces. Focus on your strengths and how you can achieve your goals. It may be okay to be motivated by the work of others but it should not stress you out. In the end, the entrance to medical school is based on simple criteria: achieve the necessary grades at A-levels, attain good scores in UCAT, and perform well in the interviews. Just focus on these goals and how you can achieve them with your own strengths.

Stress can be good for you

A minimal amount of stress can be good to motivate you to keep track of your plans. However, the way you react to stress is what matters with regard to the outcome.

Please remember that stress is nothing to be frightened of, and is inevitable. Learning how to cope with it is important to enter medical school successfully.

Hobbies, sports, and social activities

This was discussed in the previous chapter (Chapter 21). It is vital that you make sufficient time for activities outside of academic subjects to have a good study–life balance. If this is not done, you can easily become stressed out.

Make sure that you find time to do things that you enjoy, even if you are very busy preparing for A-levels and the medical school entrance exams.

Support network

It is important that you have good friends at school or college to whom you can talk. If stressed, try to talk to your friends or family or support network. Schools and colleges have career advisers as well as support systems; school nurses can direct you to the right support if you have any physical or mental illness.

Breathing exercises

Deep-breathing exercises can help to reduce stress levels; these exercises reduce the sympathomimetic chemicals that increase blood pressure and stress. You may have practised it many times before, using it in exams, interviews or stressful situations. Start practising as early as possible and regularly; you will see the benefits when you face stressful scenarios. There are free apps such as Breathe2relax that help with techniques and pictorial artefacts to help you practise these exercises.

Mindfulness strategies, relaxation techniques, and meditation can help if they have been practised before. There are free apps or YouTube videos which can help in this aspect.

Seek help early

If you have reached out to your friends and family and still feel stressed, seek out support early. Each GP surgery will have professional talking therapies that you can also refer yourself to. Your GP can give advice if these do not work. Getting help early will help in your future academic career and preparation for medical school. It is normal to feel stressed during the busy A-level years.

What signs should parents look for?

Parents can look for early signs of stress or burnout and get help immediately. These could include feeling tense, not sleeping well, being irritable, worrying a lot, having a headache or stomach pains, losing interest in food or eating more than normal, being negative with a low mood, and feeling hopeless about the future.

Having someone to talk to will help; this could be from a parent or teacher or student support centre staff or a study buddy. If you can share your worries, it helps to de-stress and recover soon. Parents should talk to their child and be involved as much as possible.

Parent support during exams

Parents know that it is a stressful time for their child during the exams or interviews or UCAT tests; they should try to be flexible during exam time. If your child is busy working hard near exam time, try not to worry about undone household jobs or leaving the bedroom untidy. Any challenging conversation can escalate the stress levels for both the student and the parent. Try to understand their emotions and help them proactively. Exams are not forever, and see if you can postpone discussing problems after exams if it is possible and appropriate. Avoid any criticism towards them during these difficult times.

Parents should tell their child that feeling anxious is normal during exams or interviews. They should motivate them by telling them that they have worked hard and encourage them to be confident. Reassure them and tell them that failing exams or interviews is not the end of the world.

Talking to your child about what went well in the exams could help; ask them in general rather than focusing too deeply on any particular question. Ask them to move on and focus on the next exam, as what has been done already cannot be changed.

Looking after your friends

It is important that you keep looking after your friends too. Listen to your friends and ask if everything is OK with them. Spending time together, staying in touch, and having social time are good and necessary. If you find that your friend is stressed, help them to get the right help. If a friend does not want to discuss medical school preparation, and says that they are worried, take it seriously and ask them if there is anything else that you can do to help. Simple words of enquiry and taking care of others will go a long way in preventing the escalation of mental health problems.

Key Points

- **A-level and medical school preparations can be stressful and daunting; taking care of your mental health is vital.**
- **Managing a routine and effective time management can avoid stress at the last minute.**
- **Be positive and avoid negative beliefs.**
- **Deep-breathing exercises can effectively help during stressful situations.**
- **Parents can support children effectively during A-levels if they adopt the right approach.**
- **Take care of your friends and look after each other.**

References

1. Google Play. Defense Health Agency. Breathe2Relax. Available from: https://play.google.com/store/apps/details?id=mil.dha.breathe2relax&hl=en_GB&pli=1.
2. GOV.UK. Ofqual. Coping with exam pressure — a guide for students. May 2025. Available from: https://www.gov.uk/government/publications/coping-with-exam-pressure-a-guide-for-students/coping-with-exam-pressure-a-guide-for-students.
3. NHS. Help your child beat exam stress. Available from: https://www.nhs.uk/mental-health/children-and-young-adults/advice-for-parents/help-your-child-beat-exam-stress/.
4. UCAS. Managing exam stress. Learn how to support your mental health during stressful periods such as exams. Available from: https://www.ucas.com/money-and-student-life/student-life/mental-health-and-wellbeing/managing-exam-stress.